By David Zinczenko

Eat This, Not That! The No-Diet Weight-Loss Solution

Eat This, Not That! For Kids

Eat This, Not That! Supermarket Survival Guide

Eat This, Not That! Restaurant Survival Guide

Eat This, Not That! Best (& Worst) Foods in America!

Cook This, Not That! Kitchen Survival Guide

Cook This, Not That! Skinny Comfort Food

Cook This, Not That! Easy & Awesome 350-Calorie Meals

Grill This, Not That! Backyard Survival Guide

Drink This, Not That! Sip Your Way to a Flat Belly!

Eat This, Not That! No-Diet Diet

The 8-Hour Diet

The New Abs Diet

The New Abs Diet for Women

The New Abs Diet Cookbook

The Abs Diet Eat Right Every Time Guide

The Abs Diet Get Fit, Stay Fit Plan

The Abs Diet Ultimate Nutrition Handbook

The Abs Diet 6-Minute Meals for 6-Pack Abs

Men, Love & Sex: The Complete User's Guide for Women

Eat It to Beat It!

ZERO
BELLY
DIET

ZERO
BELLY
DIET

DAVID ZINCZENKO

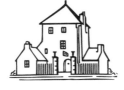

Ballantine Books
New York

Published in the United States by Ballantine Books,
an imprint of Random House, a division of Random House LLC,
a Penguin Random House Company, New York.

BALLANTINE and the HOUSE colophon are registered trademarks
of Random House LLC.

Some content adapted from the EAT THIS, NOT THAT! book series,
by David Zinczenko with Matt Goulding.

Library of Congress Cataloging-in-Publication Data
Zinczenko, David.
Zero belly diet : the revolutionary new plan to turn off your fat
genes and help keep you lean for life! / David Zinczenko
pages cm
Includes index.
ISBN 978-0-345-54795-8 (hardback)—ISBN 978-0-345-54797-2 (ebook)
1. Reducing diets. 2. Weight loss. I. Title.
RM222.2.Z565 2014
613.2'5—dc23
2014036122

Photography by Beth Bischoff

Printed in the United States of America on acid-free paper

www.ballantinebooks.com

9 8 7 6

Book design by George Karabotsos

To the researchers, scientists,
medical doctors, and other professionals
working hard to solve the riddle of obesity.
Our understanding and hope grow
every year thanks to your dedication.

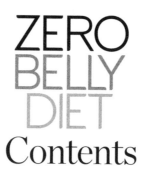

ZERO BELLY DIET

Contents

PART TWO: The Zero Belly Diet

INTRODUCTION

magine taking off your shirt, looking into the mirror, and seeing zero belly.

Not a little belly. Not a tiny bit of belly. Not a pooch or a muffin top or a spare tire or a gut.

Zero belly. A flat, rippled stomach where the softness used to be.

Most of us have long abandoned that ideal. We've accepted belly fat as an inevitable albatross, a companion for life, just a normal part of being a normal human being.

Zero belly? That's for the folks on the cover of *People* magazine, the ones with the personal trainers and the personal nutritionists and the personal liposuction machines in the basements of their Beverly Hills mansions. Ordinary folks like you and me? We'll always suffer from self-consciousness when we have to strip down to our swimsuits, always feel a little dissatisfied with the paunch around our waists, always be a little more likely to suffer the health consequences of unwanted weight gain. That's just the way it is.

But that's not true. We don't have to live that way.

As the nutrition and wellness editor for ABC News, the editorial director of *Men's Fitness*, and the former head of *Men's Health*, *Women's Health*, and *Prevention* magazines, I've spent my entire career learning about belly fat: where it comes from, what it does to us, and how we can fight back. I've literally traveled the globe reporting on fat—from launching fitness and nutrition magazines in Europe and Africa to covering the habits of Olympic athletes in Beijing. So I might just know more about your belly than anyone else on the planet.

And what I know is this: there is no greater threat to you and your family—to your health, your happiness, even your financial future—than the dumpy bit of fat that has climbed up onto your lap and nestled itself against your belly. It's a torpedo aimed at your torso, a missile fired at your midsection. It is a living, growing organism whose goal is to ruin your life.

And I've designed the ultimate program for making it disappear.

Zero belly: that's the goal.

Here's the plan.

THE ZERO BELLY PROMISE

If I were a wise, grizzled guru sitting on the top of a mountain in the Himalayas, and you traveled halfway around the globe to seek my wisdom, you'd probably be surprised by what I told you. My one secret for a better life—a healthier, wealthier, happier life—isn't "Spend more time with your friends," "Do what you love," "Find your higher power," or even "Put more money in your 401(k)." It's this: "Lose your belly." Because when it comes to physical, emotional, financial, and spiritual well-being, belly fat is more damaging to you than you would ever think.

Belly fat—what scientists call "visceral fat"—is the most dangerous fat there is: dangerous to your heart, dangerous to your brain, dangerous to your love life, and even dangerous to your wallet. The billions of enemy cells in your belly are nastier than anything the conspirators on *Homeland* could dream up—and just as dedicated to our demise. Understanding them—where they come from, what they do, and how to fight back against them—may be the most important piece of health and fitness information you will ever have.

The science proving a link between belly fat and an overall decline in personal health has only grown stronger over the last decade, and the research is clear. If you let that fat stay there, nestled on your lap, growing and making you sicker, there is no doubt about the consequences: You will live fewer years (and fewer happy years), and you will drain your savings combating the damage belly fat does to your health and well-being.

But there is an answer, a way to change your destiny and live a longer, leaner, happier life. And you're holding it in your hands.

That's the promise of ZERO BELLY, the first program to reduce belly fat dramatically, not through traditional calorie-restrictive weight-loss methods, but by actually "turning off" your fat genes and putting an end to the inflammation that causes them to switch back on.

Your genes are your genes, and that can't be changed. But how those genes express themselves can be. As Alfredo Martinez, Ph.D., professor of food sciences and nutrition at the Department of Physiology and Nutrition at the University of Navarra in Spain, most eloquently puts it, your personal genetic code "is like the lyrics of a song. You can't change the lyrics, but you can change the way the song is played—the speed, the rhythm, and the volume—by changing your diet." (Leave it to a European to make belly fat sound like opera.) If your fat genes are blasting away like Metallica, this plan can turn them down to Mozart.

And the results will be fast, measurable, and long-lasting. In a mere six weeks, you will lose as much as 7 inches off your waist

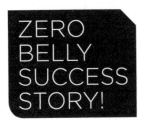

MARTHA CHESLER, *52*
Lost 21 pounds and 7 inches in six weeks

"It was great to know major health improvements were happening I couldn't even see!"

For years the Ohio teacher dabbled in diets—Medifast, Slim-Fast, Curves—but found them restrictive, hard to follow, and energy draining. **ZERO BELLY** made weight loss easy. Free to forget calorie counting and measuring, Martha was able to stop obsessing about her goal—and start dropping pounds with ease. "I saw results immediately," she reports. "I felt better physically and emotionally and wanted to keep that feeling going." And she did. In less than six weeks on the program Martha dropped over 20 pounds and an astonishing 7 inches from her middle. But the best news was about her heart health. Before starting **ZERO BELLY,** her heart rate would typically soar to 112 beats per minute (bpm) within moments of starting her exercise bike workout. "After the first week and a half I had lost 10 pounds and with the same workout I could not raise my heart rate over 96 bpm. It was great to know good things were happening that I couldn't even see."

and slash your statistical risk of dying from diabetes, heart disease, or stroke by as much as 80 percent. Consider the story of Martha Chesler on the previous page, and her journey to ZERO BELLY.

As your fat-storage genes go silent, I'll show you how to measure your improving health just as you measure your shrinking belly, using new technology that will give you the most accurate picture ever of the state of your personal well-being.

This new science is the foundation of ZERO BELLY. The ZERO BELLY foods and ZERO BELLY drinks are calibrated to disarm your fat genes, alter your genetic destiny, and reverse the march of diabetes and obesity. A 2013 study published in the *Journal of Physiology and Biochemistry* found that even after eating a high-fat, high-sugar diet—and gaining the weight and abdominal fat that comes with it—switching to a healthy eating plan can reverse the genetic changes induced by the unhealthy diet in just ten weeks.

Imagine that: a plan that can strip away a dozen or more pounds in two weeks and alter your genetic destiny in less than twelve!

A PERSONAL WEIGHT-LOSS JOURNEY

I'm passionate about the benefits of ZERO BELLY, not only because of the impact it's had on other people's lives but also because it's made such a difference in my own life as well. See, I wasn't always what you'd call healthy or fit. I came of age in the 1980s, just as the obesity crisis started to expand, and I expanded with it.

They called it the "Big Eighties" because everything was suddenly getting bigger—the hair was bigger, the shoulder pads were bigger, and, most important, the food was bigger. In 1980,

7-Eleven introduced the Big Gulp and Hershey's came out with the first king-size version of its chocolate bars. Two years later, Coca-Cola bought Columbia Pictures and started placing its drinks and food products into all of its movies.

At the same time, McDonald's started to ask, "Would you like to supersize that?" and every time, I said, "You bet!" By the time I was 14, I had 212 pounds of oily adolescent adiposity on my growing 5'10" frame. And I wasn't alone: the USDA's Economic Research Service estimates that daily calorie intake per person increased by 24.5 percent, or about 530 calories, between 1970 and 2000.

Sure, I felt bad about being fat. Sure, I was made fun of. Sure, I had trouble making friends and getting dates. My weight got so bad that the coach of our high school wrestling team recruited me to literally sit on people at the end of matches. But whenever life got me down, I had a reliable friend waiting just inside the pantry door. All I had to do was rip open another bag of Doritos and drown myself in fluorescent orange goodness, or bum a ride to the mall and follow my nose to Friendly's. Food was my refuge from feeling bad.

But deep down, I knew this wasn't the way to live. I knew I looked bad. I knew I felt bad. What I didn't know was that if I didn't change, I was headed toward physical, emotional, and even financial disaster.

It took a tragedy to wake me up.

HOW FAT HIT ME IN THE GUT

At the still-young age of 52, my father passed away from a sudden, massive stroke. Always heavy since the time I was born, he had ballooned into obesity in the 1980s in much the same way I had. I was his son. I carried the same "fat genes" that he did. Would this be my fate, too?

While I'd already begun fighting back—going through basic training in the Navy and running marathons during my early twenties—the threat of obesity was always weighing on my mind, even before my father's stroke. I trained hard, every single day, to keep the weight off, and I liked how I looked; I just didn't want to have to run 26.2 miles in order to get there.

I knew that being a marathon runner or an obsessive exerciser wasn't how I wanted to live my life. Yes, I still enjoy working out every day, but there's a great big world out there to explore, and it's hard to see it all when sweat is constantly dripping into your eyes.

More important, my father's death woke me up to the fact that excess weight—especially excess belly fat—was more than just a vanity issue. Belly fat may be the number-one cause of heart disease, stroke, diabetes, and cancer in America, and it contributes mightily to our epidemics of Alzheimer's, depression, and even inflammatory and autoimmune diseases. Indeed, new studies show that belly fat is utterly different from other types of fat. It evolves out of a different set of stem cells than the fat found in other parts of our bodies, its actions triggered by fat-storage genes that get turned on and cranked to high volume by our fast-food, high-stress lifestyle. Once those genes get turned on, visceral fat acts like an invading force, trying to take over our bodies.

What was clear to me was this: belly fat killed my dad.

I was going to find a way to fight back.

TAKING AIM AT THE ENEMY

That's how my odyssey to find a cure for belly fat began.

Ten years ago, I wrote a best-selling book called *The Abs Diet,* which launched a revolution in the way diets were built.

The Abs Diet was the first book to fully explain how muscle-building foods that were rich in protein and fiber and high in nutrients—the very foods that build abs—were also critical weapons against belly fat. And it explained how "going on a diet" was the worst thing you could do if you wanted to lose weight.

Seven years ago, I launched the Eat This, Not That! series, which showed how we could lose dramatic amounts of weight by eating all our favorite foods from the most popular restaurant chains and fast-food vendors in America. It grew to more than a dozen books, and it made a lot of food marketers angry—I got more "stop or we'll sue" letters than I care to count—but in the end, the food industry realized the only way to deal with the coming tide of consumer awareness was to get with the program.

ZERO SACRIFICE!

To me, ZERO BELLY *is an indulgence; it's a celebration of tasty, wonderful, colorful, healthy foods. I'm feeling very spoiled!*

—JUNE CARON, 55, *who lost 12 pounds in fourteen days*

Both *The Abs Diet* and *Eat This, Not That!* helped millions of Americans lose tens of millions of pounds and changed the way we eat today. Thanks to the greater awareness of hidden calories and additives in our food, restaurant chains all across the country bowed to public and government pressure and started posting their nutritional contents on websites and in their stores. One result: we've actually tapped the brakes on the march of obesity. In 2013, for the first time since government agencies have tracked these trends, the Centers for Disease Control reported a decline in childhood obesity among underprivileged kids. Nineteen states showed measurable declines; the vast majority of other states showed no increase, after decades of rising obesity rates.

But this war is only partly won.

Much of the research on belly fat that informed those earlier books was in its beginning stages. We knew that visceral fat—the fat that's underneath your stomach muscles, wrapped around your internal organs—has biochemical functions that damage the human body, almost like a parasite intent on killing its host. But we knew little about how it operates, how it creates those chemicals, and what exactly they do to us. Until now.

Today, we know that fat storage is triggered, in great part, by a series of markers in our individual genetic codes. Some of us carry a number of genes linked to metabolic disorders like diabetes and obesity; others have a lower genetic propensity for these health issues. Once the "on" switch is flipped for our fat genes, we are at risk for weight gain and all the health issues that surround it—and no amount of exercise or calorie restriction is going to reverse that course completely. (That's why so many people who diet and work out like crazy still can't lose weight! Eureka!) And the number-one trigger for our fat genes is diet—especially a lack of certain nutrients.

We've also learned more about belly fat—how it's formed, and how it behaves. A visceral fat cell is unlike any other kind of cell—fat cell or otherwise—in your body. Visceral fat doesn't even come from the same set of stem cells as other fat; it has evolved in an entirely different way. And as it gains greater purchase inside you, it spits out greater and greater levels of adipokines—a series of biochemical substances that do terrible things to your health. Adipokines raise your blood pressure, increasing your risk of stroke. They reduce your insulin sensitivity, leading to diabetes. They increase inflammation, which puts you at risk for everything from Alzheimer's to arthritis to psoriasis to cancer. They alter your hormonal response, eroding muscle tissue, increasing your risk of depression, and destroying your sex drive. They attack and scar your liver, potentially leading to cirrhosis, cancer, and ultimately liver failure.

This is what visceral fat does. This is the enemy. And it is not fooling around.

YOUR BELLY by THE NUMBERS

35 MILLION:
Number of digestive glands in your stomach

40 BILLION:
Number of visceral fat cells in the belly of the average American

100 TRILLION:
Number of bacteria in your body, about 80 percent of them in your gut

3 POUNDS:
Weight of microbes living in your digestive system

80 PERCENT:
Portion of your body's immune cells that are located in your gut

10 TIMES:
How much longer your intestinal tract is compared to your height

95 PERCENT:
Portion of serotonin, the "happiness hormone," that's located within your gut

39.7 INCHES:
Average waist circumference of the adult American man

37.5 INCHES:
Average waist circumference of the adult American woman

1.5 LITERS:
Amount of food and beverage your stomach can hold at one time.

7 SECONDS:
Time it takes for food to get from your lips to your stomach.

But in the last few years, this same research has given us several important breakthroughs—science that shows us how to finally master our midsections. And it's this new science that makes ZERO BELLY so revolutionary. In this book, you'll discover how certain foods short-circuit our fat genes—turning off the parts of our DNA that trigger weight gain and activating our bodies to burn, not store, fat. In fact, eating the right diet can essentially take your foot off the fat-gene accelerator and dramatically reverse weight gain, in the process literally changing your genetic destiny. No diet plan has ever attacked weight gain at the genetic level. ZERO BELLY does.

You'll also learn the power of proper digestion, and its role in quelling inflammation—an often-overlooked culprit in weight gain—while making us look and feel leaner and healthier. Many of the foods that form the basis of popular diets—from Shred to Atkins to Dukan to South Beach—are high in lactose (the sugar found in dairy products) and gluten (the protein found in wheat). It's true, these foods are among our best sources of muscle-building calcium and magnesium, as well as fat-burning protein and fiber. But more and more of us are discovering that we're sensitive to these ingredients, and new research has shown that even people who are not characterized as gluten-intolerant can suffer a fat-promoting inflammatory response from eating too much wheat. In fact, shocking new research has shown that the way in which we digest food and the actions of the microbes that live in our bellies can alter the action of our genes in ways that trigger us to either store or burn fat. (You had no idea you were running a microbial Holiday Inn, did you?)

As this new science has emerged—many of the relevant studies on genetics and nutrition were conducted in 2013 and 2014, and are only now reaching the research community—it's become clear that America has been racing up one side of the weight-loss hill with all of these standard diet plans, while racing back down the other side with inflammation, digestive health issues, unstoppable genetically based metabolic programming, and the eventual weight gain that ensues because none of these issues is being properly addressed. We needed a weight-loss plan that helps build muscle, burn fat, promote proper digestion, and attack belly fat at a genetic level—without exposing us to high levels of inflammatory, weight-promoting ingredients like those found in common diet plans.

That's why ZERO BELLY is so timely, so critical, and so revolutionary. ZERO BELLY is highly effective, easy, delicious, and fun to follow because it's made with real food: meats like chicken, beef, and fish; fresh fruit; even a moderate amount of chocolate. It's low in saturated fat and low in sugar (including natural sugars), provides moderate levels of protein (primarily from plants), and is high in fiber and healthy, unsaturated fats. You'll enjoy three meals and two snacks (including one delicious ZERO BELLY drink) a day, focusing primarily on plant-based foods until dinnertime. On ZERO BELLY, you'll never go hungry.

No, you won't have to measure every calorie you eat. No, you won't have to drive yourself into the ground with grueling workouts. ZERO BELLY will show you how to build a lean, strong body and strip away unwanted belly fat without those fruitless sacrifices. The result: weight loss will be easier, faster, more lasting, and (if I may say so myself) more delicious than you'd ever imagine.

THE SIMPLE PATH TO ZERO BELLY

ZERO BELLY is unlike any other diet plan ever created. It is a unique approach to weight loss that attacks belly fat in three ways:

- **First,** it lights a fire under your metabolism, triggering your body's natural calorie-burning mechanism—a mechanism that specifically targets belly fat. ZERO BELLY unleashes the power of protein, fiber, and healthy fats to burn calories by encouraging lean muscle growth and maximizing the thermogenic effects of eating—meaning, the calorie-burning effect of digesting food itself. Protein, fiber, and fat require more energy to digest than simple carbs, so in effect, you'll be burning more calories by eating more great food. These three "macronutrients" will trigger your brain's natural satiation hormones to keep you feeling full while you strip junk from your diet.

- **Second,** this plan attacks inflammation throughout the body by triggering your digestive system's natural health-defense system, shrinking bloat, easing digestion, and flattening your stomach with shocking rapidity. While ZERO BELLY isn't strictly dairy-free or gluten-free, it will substantially reduce your intake of lactose (the naturally occurring sugar in dairy), gluten (the protein found in wheat), and animal-derived saturated fat, and it will eliminate inflammation-causing additives and preservatives. Meanwhile, it will fill your body with the nutritional trigger foods that allow for digestive healing, a better balance of healthy gut bacteria, and the release of naturally occurring compounds that battle inflammation and insulin resistance.

- **Third,** and most important, this program turns off your fat-storage genes by focusing on nine power food groups that are linked directly to the emerging science of nutritional genetics—the study of how nutrients in food influence gene expression. By reversing the acceleration of your fat-storage genes, ZERO BELLY completely remaps your genetic destiny, allowing your body to return to its natural, healthful state.

And because the only thing I hate more than slaving over a stove is shopping for the food to slave over, I've built a meal plan that can easily be prepped over the weekend. Once you've prepared the basics—which can all be done while watching an episode of *House of Cards*—you will be set for the coming seven days, and need only a knife and some fresh meat and produce to put the finishing touches on your meals. (If you're more adventurous in the kitchen, there are plenty of delicious recipes for you as well.)

I'm passionate about this plan because it works—so well, in fact, that I've been personally stunned by the results.

In the spring of 2014, I assembled a panel of test subjects—average men and women just like you, from all over the country—and put them on the ZERO BELLY plan for six weeks. More than fifty subjects completed the original ZERO BELLY Challenge, and their results were astonishing. They lost as much as 24 pounds and—more significantly—up to 7 inches off their waists in those six weeks. They not only lost weight; they lost visceral fat, the troublesome fat that matters most!

In the coming pages, you'll meet some of the men and women who have discovered the magic of ZERO BELLY. People like Katrina Bridges, of Bethalto, Ohio, a 30-year-old mother of four who dropped 5 inches off her waist ("It definitely works on the tummy area, and so many women need that"). But more important, when Katrina started the program, she had almost double the risk of diabetes, heart disease, and stroke as a person of standard weight. In just six weeks, she slashed her increased risk of death by 80 percent—an improvement she can not only see but accurately measure, using the new technology I'll outline in Chapter Four.

You'll also read about success stories like Bob McMicken, a food service director from Lancaster, California, whose waist size dropped from 39 inches to 33 inches in just six weeks. He lost 24 pounds without exercising and without ever feeling hungry ("I found my favorite shirt finally covered my belly again!").

And you'll hear from Bryan Wilson of Monument, Colorado, who lost 19 pounds and a remarkable 6 inches off his waist in just the first five weeks of the program ("My pants immediately fit better . . . and my biceps, triceps, and shoulders tightened up").

These people didn't just lose weight and fit into their old clothes better. Any diet can do that for you—at least temporarily. What ZERO BELLY does, by targeting belly fat, is to dramatically reduce your risk of heart disease, diabetes, stroke, cancer, and even Alzheimer's. That's what it did for our test panel—and that's what it can do for you.

ZERO BELLY unlocks the secrets of foods that provide all the essential protein, vitamins, minerals, and fiber you need to lose weight and flip your genetic triggers, while sidestepping the traditional diet mistakes that cause hunger, inflammation, and rebound weight gain. And it almost immediately reduces the bloating and digestive discomfort that not only makes you look and feel fatter but adds to the inflammation that causes long-term weight gain.

One aspect of this plan I'm most excited about is a collection of ZERO BELLY drinks—high-nutrient, high-flavor blends that you can enjoy at any time (you'll even want to serve them for dessert) but which are so packed with protein and nutrients that they will steer you and your body straight onto the weight-loss expressway. And you can make them with a blender, some protein powder, and a handful of delicious ingredients.

Plus, to speed your own attack on belly fat, I've created a special group of ZERO BELLY workouts—full-body workouts that systematically attack belly fat, without a single sit-up! (By the way, a lot of our test panel had great results without doing the workouts.)

I'm excited about this plan for a lot of reasons, but especially for these:

- ZERO BELLY **is unique:** it targets belly fat specifically, powered by the latest revolutionary research in burning fat and building muscle with a focus on gut health, anti-inflammatory foods, and tweaking your own unique genetic programming.

- ZERO BELLY **is easy:** you'll enjoy a very simple, very delicious series of easy-to-make meals and snacks based on nine simple foods that will keep you happy, healthy, and satisfied.

- ZERO BELLY **is incredibly effective.** But don't take my word for it. Scores of men and women just like you will share their personal experiences throughout this book, and help show that ZERO BELLY is the perfect path forward to a leaner, healthier, happier life!

ZERO BELLY

My plan targets the fat that matters most—visceral belly fat—through a unique nutritional approach powered by the latest revolutionary research in weight loss, digestive health, and anti-inflammatory foods that target, and turn off, your fat genes.

MEALS:

Three square meals, one ZERO BELLY drink, and one additional snack per day.

NUTRIENTS:

While ZERO BELLY is carefully balanced to give you all the essential nutrients you need to strip away fat and reveal lean, healthy muscle, you'll ask three important ZERO BELLY questions before each meal or snack:

- **Where's my protein?**
- **Where's my fiber?**
- **Where's my healthy fat?**

FOODS:

These foods have been carefully selected for their micronutrient content; in fact, most have been linked to genetic triggers within the human genome that are associated with weight gain and metabolic disorders. They will help reset your body's genetic destiny while decreasing inflammation and attacking visceral fat with almost surgical precision.

Z ero Belly Drinks (90-second nutrition!)

E ggs

R ed fruits

O live oil and other healthy fats

B eans, rice, oats, and other healthy fiber

E xtra plant protein

L eafy greens, green tea, and bright vegetables

L ean meats and fish

Y our favorite spices and flavors (ginger, cinnamon, even chocolate)

AT A GLANCE

LIMIT:
- processed foods
- saturated fat
- sugar
- refined grains
- wheat
- dairy
- red meat

MAXIMIZE:
- high-phytonutrient fruits and vegetables
- high-fiber, high-protein nuts, legumes, and grains
- monounsaturated and polyunsaturated fats
- omega-3 fatty acids

DRINKS:
One snack a day will be a ZERO BELLY drink, a satisfying plant-based, protein-filled smoothie.

SPECIAL DIETARY CONCERNS:
ZERO BELLY is not strictly gluten-free, dairy-free, or vegan, but I've built this program specifically with these dietary concerns in mind. ZERO BELLY dramatically reduces your exposure to gluten and dairy while boosting plant-based sources of protein. If you're searching for a gluten-free, dairy-free, or vegan diet plan, you can easily adapt ZERO BELLY to fit your needs.

ALCOHOL:
Limit alcohol to one drink per day during the initial six-week program.

EXERCISE:
To turbocharge the weight-loss effects of ZERO BELLY, I've created the ZERO BELLY workouts, a unique full-body fitness experience that builds abs while simultaneously toning your entire body. There is no other workout plan like it!

ABDOMINAL EXERCISE:
The ZERO BELLY workouts eliminate the need for traditional abs exercises. But if you choose to take your fitness plan to the next level, the ZERO BELLY abs workouts can lead you to even greater gains.

PART ONE

Target the Fat that Matters Most

CHAPTER ONE

WHY BEATING BELLY FAT IS HEALTH GOAL #1

Your Belly Isn't Just Sitting There, Looking Sloppy. It's Actively Trying to Harm Your Heart, Your Muscles—and Even Your Brain!

Any diet plan can promise you weight loss. What ZERO BELLY offers you is something more: the power to wield food as a weapon, to turn off your fat genes, boost your metabolism, rebalance your gut health, and burn off fat for good.

ZERO BELLY is about putting your hand firmly on the tiller and turning hard to starboard, steering your life away from the twin icebergs of obesity and illness and out into the open water of a better destiny.

I'm not telling you that ZERO BELLY is the only way to lose weight. There are thousands of different ways you could achieve weight loss: exercise programs, calorie-restrictive diets, "master cleanses," even hypnosis. You could have surgery, you could check yourself into a clinic, you could subsist on nothing but grapefruit or peanut butter or mung beans. You could become a Weight Watcher, a Tough Mudder, a Bowflexer, a CrossFitter, a South Beacher, a Dukanite. You can Zumba, you can Shred, you can Spartan Up, you can P90X to your heart's content. They will all help you get fitter and drop a few pounds.

But they will not do what ZERO BELLY does: set a bull's-eye on the fat cells that matter most, and go at them with high-intensity, almost surgical precision until your physical, mental, and emotional health is fully restored.

AND NOW, WE INTERRUPT THIS BOOK FOR A WORD FROM OUR SPONSOR:

Hey there, friend! Do you want awesome abs of steel, delts of diamonds, buns of tungsten? Do you want to get ripped, shredded, cut, buffed, and/or filleted all over? Do you want to strip away flab and get hot-hot-hot in just weeks? Then ZERO BELLY *is for you! Act now! Order today!*

So look . . . I'm not going to downplay it. The physical transformations that ZERO BELLY can bring about are stunning. Dropping the weight equivalent of a two-year-old boy in just six weeks will change the way people look at you, and the way you look at yourself.

And if appealing to your vanity is what it takes to get you to take the first steps toward a new life, then I'm all for it. After all, studies show that vanity works—in the short term: If I told you that you were going to appear on national television in a swimsuit, and you had six weeks to get ready for it, believe me, you'd be pretty motivated to start eating differently and to stick to it.

But ZERO BELLY is more than just another weight-loss program. This plan blasts belly fat from the inside by dramatically reducing bloating and inflammation; shrinks it from the outside by melting away fat and replacing it with lean, firm muscle; and keeps attacking it on a long-term basis by turning off your genetic weight-gain switches and restoring your metabolism to what it ought to be. This three-part strategy is how my program will give you back the health you need and the happiness you deserve.

To fully grasp how virulent belly fat is, and how to fight back, it's important to understand where it comes from—and why, exactly, it behaves in the ways that it does.

KNOW THE ENEMY

A little bit of fat does a lot of good in our bodies—especially if it's located in exactly the right places. It helps to keep us warm in winter and stores energy for later use. It's involved in some important chemical reactions as well. A shapely little bit of fat produces the hormone leptin, which travels to the hypothalamus, the part of the brain that controls appetite, and flicks the switch that tells us to stop eating. It also produces adiponectin, another hormone that helps regulate the metabolism of lipids and blood sugar. In fact, in a 2014 study published in the journal *Cell Metabolism,* researchers reported that subcutaneous fat in your hips and thighs is associated with reduced insulin levels and increased insulin sensitivity (meaning that it actually protects against diabetes). People who are "pear-shaped" and store fat in their hips and thighs also tend to have higher HDL cholesterol (the good kind) and lower triglycerides, which means that Kim Kardashian may live *forever*.

But biologically, there's an enormous difference between subcutaneous fat—the stuff that's right below your skin, the stuff that makes up love handles and the like—and visceral fat, which is inside your abdominal wall, wrapped around your internal organs. The easiest way to tell the difference might be this: subcutaneous fat jiggles, but visceral fat doesn't. Subcutaneous fat is fat you can pinch; visceral fat is the solid stuff that makes your gut stick out. Subcutaneous fat comes in different colors (white, brown, and beige), each of which has some positive health benefits. (To learn more about the oddly complex world of fat, check out "Fifty Shades of Fat" on page 46.)

But unlike its subcutaneous cousin, visceral fat isn't just hanging out, keeping us warm. It's more like an active volcano. It's spewing out dangerous substances all the time.

Indeed, visceral fat secretes more than a hundred biochemicals, which are collectively known as adipokines. But they ought to be known as adipo-unkinds, because they include such nasty substances as:

- **Resistin,** a hormone that undermines your body's ability to metabolize glucose and leads to high blood sugar

- **Angiotensinogen,** a compound that raises blood pressure

- **Interleukin-6,** a chemical associated with arterial inflammation

- **Tumor necrosis factor**, which is as bad as it sounds—it causes inflammatory issues such as psoriasis, Crohn's disease, and various forms of arthritis

And the more visceral fat you have, the less of the positive fat-based substances (like adiponectin) your body seems to be capable of producing. In fact, increased visceral fat can be a sign that your subcutaneous fat is not functioning properly, according to research by Michael Jensen, M.D., of the Endocrine Research Unit at the Mayo Clinic. That may explain why more visceral fat equals less positive fat-based adiponectin. Decreased adiponectin is linked to increased risk of type 2 diabetes, elevated glucose levels, hypertension, cardiovascular disease, and even some types of malignancies, according to the National Institutes of Health.

Visceral fat also increases the amount of estrogen in your body, and interferes with the function of your liver, meaning your body has a harder time flushing away toxins—including the very toxins that fat is creating! In fact, visceral fat does the same thing to your liver that chronic alcoholism does; a recent study at the Mayo Clinic found that one in ten cases of liver failure resulting in the need for a liver transplant is now caused by nonalcoholic steatohepatitis, or NASH—a newly coined term for liver damage caused by visceral fat.

You can think of having belly fat as being in a state of chronic inflammation—your body is being irritated and attacked, 24/7, by the substances your belly fat spews out. For some reason, men are much more likely than women to store fat in their midsections, although plenty of women have this "apple shape" as well. And new research is showing that children may be even more vulnerable: 10 percent of children in the United States may already have liver damage caused by visceral fat, according to federal surveys.

But removing that visceral fat—which is exactly what ZERO BELLY is designed to do—helps to remove those risks.

THE ALIEN INSIDE YOU

So stop thinking of belly fat as a (literal) extension of your fine self, and start thinking of it as what it really is—a living, squirming parasite inside your body that's out to ruin your life.

I know. Gross. But true.

This visceral-fat creature wrapped around your internal organs is eager to grow and cause even more mischief. And we now know that there are three specific factors that contribute to the growth of visceral fat: a diet low in fiber, high in carbs and high in saturated fat; chronic inflammation; and a genetic propensity toward visceral fat storage that's been triggered by the previous two factors. Once your fat storage system is turned on, you're set up for a bigger belly. I'll explain more about fat genes and how to turn them off in the next chapter, but before I do, I want to outline more about why it's so important to focus on belly fat.

Every time you take in more energy than you burn off, the individual visceral fat cells inside your body become larger. The larger the fat cells, the more metabolically active they are. And activated fat cells have one goal in life: to make themselves even bigger. So they send out adipokines to cause more inflammation, which helps shut down your satiation hormones, which makes you crave more carbs and saturated fat, which you then eat, causing more fat storage and giving your belly fat even more power. Your belly fat basically tricks you into helping it grow.

But as fat cells become more metabolically active, they also become more toxic. So each time your weight goes up a single percentage point, your health risk goes up a lot more. When you accumulate visceral fat, you begin showing signs of something scientists call "metabolic syndrome." Metabolic syndrome is a condition that's really just a collection of heart disease risk factors: a larger waist, high triglycerides (the fat in your blood), high blood sugar, low HDL cholesterol, and high blood pressure. This combination increases the likelihood that you'll

- **Develop diabetes:** 500 percent increase

- **Have a heart attack:** 300 percent increase

- **Die of a heart attack:** 200 percent increase

Recent estimates are that between ages 20 and 39, about 16 percent of women and 17 percent of men are already in the throes of metabolic syndrome; between ages 40 and 59, about 37 percent of women and more than 40 percent of men are; and by the time we hit 60, a majority of us all are symptomatic. In fact, visceral fat has been linked to pretty much every epidemic of our modern times, including not just diabetes and heart disease but high blood pressure, colon cancer, breast cancer, and prostate cancer. (It is also a major contributor to the relentless spread of "mom jeans.")

Think about it for a moment: Heart disease. Diabetes. Cancer.

How many loved ones have you lost to those three devils? How many times have you worried that one of the devils was hunting you? How many doctor's appointments have you rushed to—or put off going to—because you thought that cough, that pain, that dizzy feeling meant one or more of those health problems might have you in its grasp? And how much are you already spending on medication to keep them at bay?

Now consider that I've seen ZERO BELLY reduce the risk of death from obesity-related disease in just six weeks—by up to 80 percent in at least one of our participants.

Like I said, any weight-loss plan can help you lose a few pounds. But ZERO BELLY is specifically designed to target the fat that matters most to your health: visceral fat—the kind that insinuates its way in and around your internal organs. Visceral fat is a living, breathing welcome committee for disease.

I'll go much more into the science of this later in this book, but recent and ongoing studies have found that just carrying around extra weight isn't necessarily the worst thing that can happen to your health. Where and how fat is distributed in your body makes all the difference. In fact, belly fat alone may be the number-one contributor to three of the biggest killers of our modern times. According to a Mayo Clinic study of 650,000 adults, greater waist circumference means greater risk of death at pretty much every turn.

In a study presented in fall 2013 to the American Heart Association, researchers reported following 972 obese people over eight years. They found that those who store most of their fat just beneath the skin—subcutaneous fat—were not at increased risk for heart disease, no matter how much they weighed or how broad their waistlines. But patients with high levels of visceral fat were much more likely to develop heart disease, including heart attacks, strokes, heart failure, and atrial fibrillation (irregular heartbeat).

High levels of belly fat are also linked directly to diabetes risk. In a trial that followed participants for more than eight years, researchers tracked two sets of people who had recently been diagnosed with type 2 diabetes. One set followed a low-fat diet, while the second group followed a diet high in the fruits, vegetables, lean proteins, and healthy fats that make up the ZERO BELLY plan. Those in the second group went significantly longer before needing diabetes medication, and more of them had their diabetes go into remission.

Most people understand that heart disease and diabetes are linked to weight gain. But more and more scientific research is finding a direct link between visceral fat and a variety of cancers, especially prostate, breast, and colon cancer. And in a recent paper, Italian researchers outlined how they have begun to study adipokines as markers for autoimmune diseases like rheumatoid arthritis. In the near future, doctors may be able to predict whether you'll get everything from arthritis to irritable bowel syndrome to psoriasis and even Alzheimer's by measuring how active your visceral fat is. Imagine that: we may soon be able to tell exactly how much mental decline you'll suffer based on how effective your belly fat is at attacking your brain. Makes you want to attack the fat first, right?

And if that doesn't make your head reel, then grab hold of your cerebellum, because this will blow your mind. Visceral fat tries to grow itself not just by messing with your hormones and making you more hungry but also by killing off other parts of your body, particularly your muscles.

Let me say that again: like a parasite, visceral fat literally kills off other parts of your body to keep itself alive.

I know what you're thinking: "Fire up that liposuction machine and let's hoover this monster out of me now!" Unfortunately, it doesn't work like that. Because visceral fat literally wraps itself around your liver and other vital organs, there's no way to safely remove it with surgery. There's only one viable answer.

Fortunately, you're holding the key in your hands.

WHY WE MUST MUSCLE OUT FAT

Cutting out the fat isn't possible. Cutting down on calories and starving yourself isn't going to work, either. Here's why.

One of the best ways to protect yourself against visceral fat is to strengthen and protect your muscles. Muscle burns energy on a regular basis, so it steals energy away from fat cells—specifically visceral fat cells—in order to sustain itself. Unlike, say, a sprint through the airport, which requires an instant burst of energy, muscle draws down on your fat banks slowly, like a hidden service fee. In fact, pound for pound, muscle burns about three times as many calories as fat does, just hanging out.

Plus, muscles do something else visceral fat hates: muscles store energy. When you lift a bag of groceries, go for a bike ride, or flee an invading zombie apocalypse, your muscles quickly burn up energy that they've got stored (in the form of glycogen). After you're done lifting, biking, or fleeing, your fat-storage hormones are subdued because your body wants to use any incoming calories to restore the depleted glycogen in your muscle that you burned up during exercise. So building muscle, and working that muscle, robs visceral fat of the ability to grow larger.

If you're a visceral fat cell parasite and you want to get bigger and eat up more space so you can send out more harmful adipokines, what do you want to do? You want to erode the body's muscle. And that's what makes visceral fat so damn tricky.

When people panic and decide they want to lose fat fast, they go on crash diets, restricting calories and doubling down on aerobics classes. Unfortunately, the one thing that crash dieting does very effectively is erode muscle. As I outlined above, muscle eats up energy. So when your body doesn't get enough energy, it would rather shed all that calorie-sucking muscle tissue than get rid of visceral fat. In fact, one recent study that got a lot of attention in early 2014 was conducted by Swedish and Spanish researchers, in which they put men on a diet of 360 calories a day (that's about the equivalent of half a Whopper) and made them exercise for nearly nine hours a day for four days. The men lost an average of 11 pounds. Victory!

Except this is exactly the kind of short-term victory that

leads to long-term defeat. The majority of the weight the men lost wasn't fat, it was muscle. And that's a great recipe for more visceral fat. That's why spending a month on rice cakes or doing a Master Cleanse will, in the long run, just add to the foul ranks of your belly's invading horde. (There is, however, a way to do a short-term cleanse as part of the overall ZERO BELLY plan; an effective 7-day solution is in Chapter Eleven.)

That's how I'd like you to think of visceral fat: it's an invading army, and it's literally trying to kill off your defenses, using those above-mentioned adipokines. Among the many things adipokines do is to decrease your ability to store energy, which further damages your body's ability to regulate blood sugar. In a 2009 report by the Canadian government, researchers reported that gaining a few pounds can result in almost instant damage to your muscles: "This development can be very rapid (i.e., within days), and precedes the increase in lipid uptake and accumulation that leads to insulin resistance."

And if you know about the importance of strong muscles, you know about the importance of strong bones, and how the two are interconnected. In a recent report out of Columbia University, researchers found that women with the most visceral fat had about 30 percent lower bone volume and greater bone brittleness and porosity than those women with the least amount of visceral fat.

This is why I wrote *Zero Belly Diet*, and why I believe we should all stop worrying about our weight and start targeting the fat that matters most. In the coming chapters, you'll begin doing just that.

THE AMAZING ZERO BELLY BENEFITS

Shrinking your waist by up to six inches, and dropping the equivalent of a bowling ball in weight, in just six weeks is going to make an enormous difference in the way people look at you, and in the way you look at yourself. But my goal has always been something more than just vanity. ZERO BELLY can bring you more than just, well, ZERO BELLY. It can also bring you . . .

ZERO BRAIN DRAIN!

As a kid, I often thought people took me less seriously because I was overweight. Turns out I was probably right. Overweight people often suffer from the prejudice that they're not as bright as their more slender and nimble peers. But there's a scary truth underlying that prejudice.

While greater weight and lower intelligence don't go hand in hand, over time being heavier will damage your brain. For years, scientists have understood that midlife obesity is a risk factor for dementia later in life. Just as belly fat helps cause the formation of plaque in your coronary arteries, so too does it clog up the arteries feeding the brain—a contributing factor in the develop-

IT'S A BIG, BIG, BIG, BIG WORLD!

If you sometimes feel like America's bellies have gotten out of control, you're right.

Nearly 10 percent of all American medical dollars is now spent on obesity. That means the bigger your pants, the emptier your pockets. But it's also an economic drain on all of us, including the lean; everything from our insurance costs to our airline ticket prices are increasing, thanks to obesity. Step aside and make way, because we need extra room for our new . . .

ment of Alzheimer's. According to researchers at Rush University Medical Center, the protein responsible for metabolizing fat in the liver is the same protein found in the hippocampus, the part of the brain that controls memory and learning. People with higher levels of abdominal fat actually have depleted levels of this fat-metabolizing protein, making them 3.6 times more likely to suffer from memory loss and dementia later in life.

But a few years ago, scientists discovered something even more ominous. They performed CT scans on a number of healthy, middle-aged men and women to measure their visceral fat. What they learned was that the more visceral fat a person had, the less brain mass they had.

ZERO LIABILITY!

Weight gain costs us a lot of money—and not just in ripped pant seams and popped skirt buttons. In fact, obese men spend on average an additional $6,518 more in annual health care costs

BIGGER BUSES

The Federal Transit Administration wants to raise the assumed average weight of bus passengers from 150 to 175 pounds "to acknowledge the expanding girth of the average passenger," according to the *New York Times.*

BIGGER BOSOMS

At Wacoal America, one of the largest bra makers in the country, 36DD recently became its most popular size. As recently as 2006, it was 36C.

BIGGER BOATS

The Coast Guard now says that fewer of us can fit on standard-size boats, and it's increased the assumed average weight per person to 185 pounds.

continued

than normal-weight men. For women, the burden is even greater: they fork over an additional $8,365 in potbelly penalties each year. In fact, by one estimate, obesity-related health care will cost Americans $190 billion this year alone.

Recently, Duke University looked at seventeen thousand of its employees to see how their weight impacted their health care costs. The results? Well, let's just say that the more pounds you pack on, the greater the shadow you cast on your financial future. In fact, for each one-unit uptick in body mass index (BMI) above 19—the low end of healthy weight—a man's medical costs increased by 4 percent and his drug costs increased by 2 percent. Which says a lot, since the average American man's BMI is 26.6. (The average woman's: 26.5.)

But the real cost of being overweight doesn't come in the form of prescription pills and diet products. It's not the money we spend on obesity; it's the money that obesity prevents us from making.

In a study published in the *International Journal of Obesity*,

IT'S A BIG, BIG, BIG, BIG WORLD continued

BIGGER YOUNG PEOPLE

"Overall only 1 in 4 of our young adults between the ages of 17 and 24 is eligible for military service," according to a study by the military. Obesity is the main cause.

BIGGER VERY, VERY YOUNG PEOPLE

One-third of infants in the United States are obese or at risk for obesity, according to a Wayne State University study.

BIGGER CATS AND DOGS

More than half of all pets now qualify as overweight or obese.

researchers gave participants a series of résumés with small photos of the applicants attached. What they learned was that starting salary, leadership potential, and hiring decisions were impacted negatively when the photo showed a person who was overweight—most severely in the case of obese women. How do the researchers know that weight was the deciding factor and not their experience or general looks? Because they used the same individuals, before and after weight-loss surgery!

And we can put real numbers against this prejudice. One study by researchers at the University of Florida found that the thinnest women make a whopping $22,283 more then their over-weight peers. For American women, gaining 25 pounds results in an average salary differential of $15,572. Think of it this way: an overweight woman who works for 25 years will wind up with $389,300 less than a thinner one. Add in 25 years of paying that extra eight grand in health care costs, and the total swing between slender and stocky amounts to $598,425.

Think dropping 25 pounds might be worth a cool 600 G's?

BIGGER MOVIE THEATERS

The average movie seat has increased from 20 inches wide to as much as 26 inches; theaters now spend nearly a third more on their building space than they did just twenty years ago. (Imagine if they put that money into actually making the movies better!)

BIGGER AMBULANCES

Boston's emergency services recently retrofitted an ambulance to make it capable of ferrying people up to 850 pounds.

BIGGER COFFINS

Goliath Casket makes models up to 52 inches wide, and they cater to those whose lives are cut short by obesity. "We sell about 300 caskets per year, and my records show the average age of the deceased is 45 or younger," says Keith Davis, the company's president.

ZERO HANG-UPS!

What's more exciting than a cold six-pack on a hot day? A hot six-pack on a cold day. And that's what ZERO BELLY can give you. But it's not just about how you'll look. It's about how terrific your sexual drive and performance will become.

You already know that a poor diet leads to high cholesterol and high blood pressure, both of which damage the circulatory system and gum up the flow of blood to your heart. Well, it does the same to your other love organs as well. And less blood flow is never a good thing, especially in the realm of romance.

And you already know that a flat, firm belly is the ultimate symbol of sexiness—which is why we all look twice when someone with a washboard stomach uses the bottom of his or her T-shirt to wipe away workout sweat.

Well, new research has discovered an even more sinister way in which belly fat, in particular, can harm your sexuality. In studies, women with visceral fat accumulation have been shown to have elevated secretions of cortisol, a stress hormone, and an increased sensitivity to stress hormones in the hypothalamus, pituitary, and adrenal glands. Cortisol makes us gain visceral fat (one more way that old devil tries to grow itself), so more visceral fat equals more cortisol, which equals more visceral fat. But worse, women who show an increase in cortisol in response to sexual stimuli report less satisfaction with their sex life compared with women who show a decrease in cortisol. Good sex comes from less stress. Abdominal fat causes more stress, which causes bad sex.

ZERO EMISSIONS!

I designed this program specifically to balance and improve the function of your digestive system. This will reduce bloating, trigger weight loss, and actually turn off certain genes that are related to weight gain and diabetes. By reversing bloating and inflammation, you'll also be noticing less aggravation in your digestive tract. (And less aggravation on the part of your partner, too.) Within a few days, you'll be running as clean as a human Tesla.

Bloating and gas aren't just embarrassing; they're symptomatic of gastric inflammation and a digestive system that's working too hard to digest foods it's not conditioned to digest. That's damaging to the "good" bacteria in your system, and it causes weight gain.

There's another sort of gastric emission I want to mention as well: gastroesophageal reflux disease, or GERD.

GERD happens when the sphincter at the top of the stomach begins to leak, and stomach acid washes up into the esophagus and burns the tender mucous membranes in the throat. That's the cause of heartburn, but it can also lead to more serious issues, including ulcers and even esophageal cancer. And a study published in the journal *Gut* found a direct link between belly fat and Barrett's esophagus, a condition that affects the lining of the esophagus and puts subjects at an advanced risk of esophageal cancer.

Obesity is one of the biggest contributors to GERD, so it makes sense that your risk will decrease as you follow the program and lose weight rapidly. But the number of test panel participants who reported dramatic reductions in GERD—many even going off medications for the first time in years—was astounding.

ZERO DARK THIRTIES!

And forties and fifties and sixties as well.

ZERO BELLY balances your gut bacteria, which might not sound related to your mental health—until you realize that more than 90 percent of our "feel good" hormone serotonin is stored in the digestive system. In a recent study, researchers in Ireland found that mice who were treated with gut-healthy bacteria suffered less stress, anxiety, and depression-related behavior.

And new research published in the British journal *Age and Ageing* indicates that losing belly fat may be the most significant thing you can do to improve your life as you get older. In a study, researchers surveyed nearly six hundred men between the ages of 60 and 74, asking them about a wide range of issues, from their physical health to their social lives to their mental and emotional well-being. Then, the researchers measured their testosterone levels and, using X-rays and MRIs, measured their visceral and subcutaneous fat levels as well. What they discovered was that the greatest single factor impacting quality of life was visceral fat—the more belly fat these men had, the more likely they were to report unhappiness in their lives.

CHAPTER TWO

TURN OFF YOUR FAT GENES!

The Incredible New Science of How Fat Genes Get Turned On and the Magic Foods That Shut Them Off!

If anyone has ever told you that you're overweight because you're lazy, they're wrong.

If they've ever told you that you're overweight because you're gluttonous and greedy and lacking in self-control, they're wrong.

If they've ever told you that there's something wrong with you as a person, that you're "eating your feelings," and that your weight is all your fault, they're wrong.

And if they've ever told you that you've inherited the fat genes and there's nothing you can do about it, they're wrong.

Your weight is not your fault. Your genetic destiny can change. And you can—you will—get slim, and stay slim for life.

Here, at last, is the proof.

A DIP IN THE GENE POOL

It's a question that's been haunting me for decades: if weight gain is just a matter of eating more calories than you burn off, and weight loss is as simple as burning off more calories than you eat, then how is it possible that weight is "genetic"? Why do some people weigh 125 pounds without ever dieting or working out, and others weigh 250 pounds despite owning every piece of exercise equipment ever invented? And why do some family members seem to inherit the fat genes (like Beau Bridges), while others manage to stay slim and win an Oscar (like Jeff Bridges)?

Sure, some people have naturally slower metabolisms. But it's not like some of us have hamster heartbeats and others have cardiac muscles that move like a sloth. We all live pretty much the same way: we pump blood, breathe air, sleep lying down, and complain about how terrible *The Real Housewives* are while watching through our splayed fingers. And yet some of us get fat and others don't.

As a child, I was told I had inherited the fat genes. As I said in the introduction to this book, my own father was terribly overweight and died of a stroke at age 52. And as a teenager, I ballooned to well over 200 pounds myself. Obviously, it was genetic. Like father, like son, and there was little I could do about it. I was doomed to a life of *Hindenburg*-like proportions.

But wait. There was one missing link in this seemingly uninterrupted chain of chunkiness: my older brother, Eric.

Eric was my hero—and my sworn enemy. As my big brother, he seemed like Superman to me. He was, and is, a terrific athlete, daring adventurer, and all-around model of fitness. And I wasn't.

Why? How come Eric—the guy who seemed to excel at every sport known to man, who won athletic scholarships to college, and who whupped my butt just about every time he could—never got the fat genes? Why did he stay slimmer and fitter (and more popular) through high school, always excelling at hockey, football, and hoops, while I seemed to be shaped a lot more like the ball than the player? Why was he able to pig out whenever he wanted and still keep getting leaner and stronger, while everything I ate went right to my belly?

"Bad genes"? Screw that. There had to be more to it.

And there is. We had the same parents. We had the same genes. The same fat genes. But one thing was different: my fat genes switched on, and his didn't.

You see, the truth about the fat genes (and there are a number of them) is that they're sort of like a loaded gun. They're totally harmless—until you pull the trigger.

DISARM THE FAT GENES

If you've ever suspected that you inherited the fat genes, if you've ever dieted and exercised and seen little if any impact, then get ready for a revolution. Some of the most exciting research of the past several years has centered on how, exactly, that trigger gets pulled—and how we can impose some gene control.

For example, recent studies have centered on how diet can turn on (or turn off) certain genes in our bodies that cause us to store fat in our abdomens, at the same time hampering insulin regulation and putting us at risk for diabetes. In a 2014 study published in the journal *Diabetes*, researchers fed a group of normal-weight young people a whole bunch of high-fat, high-calorie muffins for seven weeks. Surprise, surprise: they all gained weight.

But how they gained weight was the shocker. Those whose fatty muffins contained saturated fat—in this case, from palm oil—gained primarily abdominal fat (twice as much abdominal fat as the other group). Those whose muffins were mostly poly-unsaturated fat, from sunflower oil, gained primarily muscle

THE FAT GENE PRIMER

For generations, we've understood the concept of "the fat gene." Obesity runs in families, and if Mom and Dad are both heavy, there's little you can do about it.

But emerging science says that's not so. Nutritional genetics may be the most important breakthrough in the battle against weight gain since the invention of the treadmill. In fact, a recent presentation by Karen L. Edwards, Ph.D., director of the University of Washington Center for Genomics and Public Health, identified a series of risk factors for obesity. They included the usual suspects: high-calorie, low-nutrient diet; physical inactivity; aging; various medical conditions; even race and socioeconomic status. But two other major risk factors stand out: family history and genetic susceptibility.

For the first time, we're learning that these "inescapable" risk factors may be very escapable, indeed. And this might just be the most exciting science I've seen in two decades of exercise and nutrition research.

The study of nutritional genetics can be broken down into two aspects: nutrigenomics,

(three times as much, in fact). Why? Because of what happened to their fat genes. According to the study authors, genes involved in regulating metabolism, insulin resistance, body composition, and fat cell differentiation behaved differently in the test subjects, depending on their diet.

Let me state this another way: even if you overeat by the same amount, you'll have less body fat if you're overeating the right fats, because your fat genes won't be triggered.

Exactly as I'd always suspected. Gaining fat isn't just about how much you eat; it's about *what* you eat. My brother didn't get

---

which is the way in which foods influence gene expression generally, and nutrigenetics, which is the way an individual's gene code responds to a particular nutrient. A September 2013 report in the journal *Advanced Nutrition* describes the behavior of genes related to obesity and diabetes as "inheritable and reversible," and researchers further state that "epigenetic mechanisms are quite important in the development of transgenerational and adult obesity as well as in the development of diabetes."

While everyone's genetic makeup is unique, we've learned enough about nutrition and its impact on DNA to identify nine food groups—the ZERO BELLY foods—that influence the expression of genes related to obesity, visceral fat gain, insulin resistance, inflammation, and fatty liver

disorder—a condition directly linked to visceral fat.

These genes get "turned on" at some point in our lives—often in early childhood—by a variety of factors, primary among them a lack of proper nutrition. In simple terms, if too much of your early diet comes from Frankenberries instead of strawberries, the lack of nutrients eventually flips your switch. And the more bad food you eat, the faster those fat genes rev. But today we know that we can decelerate the action of the genes that cause obesity and diabetes, triggering dramatic weight loss that's not based on fewer calories, but on a healthy, sustainable, long-term diet plan.

For the first time, science has shown us how we can build a diet designed to attack belly fat and improve health on a genetic level. This is the core of ZERO BELLY.

the lucky genes, and he didn't pig out any less than I did—he just ate smarter. While he was more likely to snack on whole foods like fruits or whole-grain-and-protein combos like turkey sandwiches, I was the one whose fingers were always neon orange from the processed, packaged food I'd snarfed. (Lesson: if I'd just ordered differently at lunch, maybe I would have gotten the athletic scholarship instead of a boatload of student loans!)

In fact, what we're learning now is that weight gain is caused not by genetics but by epigenetics—basically, the science of how genes are turned on and off by different environmental factors, including stress, chemical exposure, and, yes, diet. A 2014 study in the journal *Advanced Nutrition* reported that obese and diabetic people have a different pattern of epigenetic markers than those who are not obese or diabetic. Simply put, their fat genes have been tripped.

"What you eat, and don't eat, can influence which genes are turned on and when," says Kevin L. Schalinske, Ph.D., professor in the Department of Food Science and Human Nutrition at Iowa State University. "Eating the wrong foods, deficiencies in the diet, and lifestyle choices like smoking, can turn things on."

There are two pieces of good news that come with this latest research. The first is that because science can tell us when these genes have become activated, it may soon be possible for us to get a simple blood test that tells us whether we're going to become obese or diabetic—and take a medication that can "disarm" those genes and reverse our fate. We may also be able to customize diets on an individual basis—to literally identify which fat genes we carry, so we know which nutrients to double down on. This field of study, called nutritional genetics, basically looks at how different foods interact with particular genes to increase or decrease the risk of diseases like obesity, heart disease, and diabetes. And what it tells us is that counting calories isn't an effective path to permanent weight loss—but eating the right way can alter everything.

FROM HUNGRY TO HAPPY

One of the clichés about overweight people is that they're always eating, digging into every bag of chips, cookie tray, and all-you-can-eat buffet with the blind frenzy of a One Direction fan at a ticket giveaway. They must be gluttonous, which is why they're always eating, which is why they're overweight. Hence it's their own fault.

But the new genetic science is blowing that prejudice right out of the water. In fact, in 2009 researchers found that a high-fat diet modified the way in which leptin—the "satiety" hormone that's produced by our fat cells—behaved inside the body. Rats that were fed higher levels of fat and calories had lower levels of leptin in their systems, and hence were less likely to feel like they'd had enough to eat.

That's pretty amazing: Eating too much causes a shift in the way our genes behave—and triggers a vicious cycle, in which the more belly fat you gain, the harder it is for you to stop eating. (Remember what I said in previous chapters: belly fat is an attacking organism inside your body, and it wants to trick you into helping it grow bigger.)

But what's even more amazing is that what your parents ate before you were born and what you ate in your first years of childhood may be making it harder for you to stop eating now, as an adult.

In fact, a study published in *Advances in Nutrition* identified

ZERO HUNGER!

We loved the burgers! My wife and I decided to add a salad to each meal; the pounds started melting off!

—KYLE CAMBRIDGE, *28, who lost 15 pounds in fourteen days*

FOODS THAT TURN OFF YOUR FAT GENES

NUTRIENT	ZERO BELLY FOOD SOURCE	TURNS OFF GENES FOR
Betaine	Brown Rice, Quinoa & Oats; Leafy Greens, Green Tea & Brightly Colored Vegetables (spinach, beets)	Insulin resistance, liver steatosis (fatty liver)
Choline	Eggs & Lean Protein (shrimp, scallops, chicken, turkey, cod, tuna, salmon, beef); Leafy Greens, Green Tea & Brightly Colored Vegetables (collard greens)	Liver steatosis
Folate	Legumes (lentils, beans); Leafy Greens, Green Tea & Brightly Colored Vegetables (asparagus, spinach)	Insulin resistance, adiposity
Methionine	Eggs & Lean Protein (halibut, orange roughy, chicken, tuna, turkey, freshwater fish, such as pike and sunfish)	Insulin resistance, obesity
Vitamin B$_{12}$	Eggs & Lean Protein (beef, salmon, tuna, cod, lamb, shellfish, sardines)	Insulin resistance, obesity
Curcumin	Yellow, Black & Brown Spices (turmeric)	Inflammation, obesity
Epigallocatechin-3-gallate	Leafy Greens, Green Tea & Brightly Colored Vegetables (green tea)	Obesity, insulin resistance, liver steatosis
Genistein	Legumes (beans, peanut butter)	Obesity
Resveratrol	Red fruits (red grapes, blueberries); Legumes (peanut butter); Yellow, Black & Brown Spices (dark chocolate)	Obesity, liver steatosis
Sulforaphane	Leafy Greens, Green Tea & Brightly Colored Vegetables (kohlrabi, kale); Yellow, Black & Brown Spices (horseradish)	Adipocyte differentiation (basically, turning a stem cell into a fat cell)
Butyrate (a fatty acid produced in your colon by bacteria feasting on fiber)	Brown Rice, Quinoa & Oats; Yellow, Black & Brown Spices (dark chocolate)	Insulin resistance, inflammation

three factors as influencing your likelihood of developing insulin resistance later in life:

- **What your mom ate**

- **Whether your mom was overweight—and hence subject to a lot of inflammation in her system**

- **How stressed out Mom was, and how that stress may have impacted her hormonal balance**

These three factors can flip the genetic switch, and from the moment you exit the womb, you may be predisposed to obesity. In a review of forty-six different studies on the topic of obesity and epigenetics, researchers writing in the *International Journal of Obesity* in 2014 reported that epigenetic markers for obesity— evidence that the fat genes have been turned on—can be spotted at birth, and those markers can predict whether a newborn will become obese as an adult.

That might sound like science fiction, but look around you. The evidence is inescapable, in our nursery schools, in our kindergartens, on our playgrounds. If you don't believe that your parents' behavior and your in-utero environment can affect your fat genes, consider this: an estimated 22 million children under the age of 5 are overweight—and it's not because they stopped going to the gym.

A 2013 report by Britain's Royal Society of Biological Sciences laid out just how our genes have gotten away from us. According to the World Health Organization, 75 percent of the adult population of the world will be overweight, and 41 percent obese. The researchers also pointed out that the number of overweight children in the United States has doubled since 1980.

But, the researchers reiterate, "several epigenetic marks are modifiable, by changing the exposure in utero, but also by lifestyle changes in adult life."

The more we learn about fat genes—and there are a num-

FIVE WAYS TO NEUTRALIZE YOUR FAT GENES

Being born with the genes for fat storage doesn't cause you to become fat. Those genes need help getting started. Here are some unexpected ways to throw a damper on your fat genes and keep them stuck in neutral for good.

1 Cut down on saturated fats and sugar

You know fat and sugar is bad for you, but what's really interesting is the new research on how they conspire with your genes to set you up for weight gain. Foods high in saturated fats seem to cause weight gain even if calorie intake stays the same. Researchers believe there's an epigenetic factor at work. The combination of sugar and fat has been dubbed an "obesogenic environment," much in the same way a toxic waste dump linked to a cancer outbreak might be referred to as a "carcinogenic environment."

2
Don't take vitamins

Increased levels of B vitamins have long been associated with a higher prevalence of obesity and diabetes. Researchers believe that fortified infant formula may trigger the fat genes. If you're more comfortable taking a daily multivitamin, it's probably fine, but megadosing may do more harm than good.

3
Be cautious of canned foods

The concern here is a compound called BPA, or bisphenol-A. Used to make plastic softer, it's found in some plastic containers and also in the thin plastic linings of food cans. Research has indicated that it may have an epigenetic effect on humans. BPA leaks into foods that are acidic or fatty, like tomatoes, tuna, and baby formula. BPA is used by most manufacturers, but Eden Organic and Trader Joe's both sell BPA-free canned goods.

4
Go for a morning walk

Bizarre but true: recent research published in the journal *PLOS ONE* found that getting direct exposure to sunlight between 8:00 a.m. and noon reduced your risk of weight gain regardless of activity level, caloric intake, or age. It's possible that morning light synchronizes your metabolism and undercuts your fat genes.

5
Cut down on antibiotics

Our gut bacteria play a big role in keeping our fat genes in check by chomping on fiber and creating short-chain fatty acids (SCFAs) such as butyrate, which you'll read more about in Chapter Two. SCFAs help tame our genetic propensity for weight gain and diabetes. When we take antibiotics for every sniffle, we create disorder in our gut bacteria and undermine their ability to create the SCFAs that keep our fat genes in check.

ber of different ones, which control insulin sensitivity, general weight, and the manner in which stem cells "decide" to become fat cells—the more we're learning that we can actually turn them off. In fact, in animal studies, researchers have been able to delete some fat genes altogether. Research at the USDA Human Nutrition Center on Aging at Tufts University looked at a gene called, appropriately, FAT10. In mouse studies, the gene seemed to be turned on by inflammation; when it was, it slowed the mice's metabolism and increased their risk for certain cancers. When the researchers turned off the gene, not only did the mice lose body fat, but their aging slowed—and their life span increased by 20 percent!

If you're having trouble losing weight, nutritional genomics may hold the answer. The key is to undo the damage by rebalancing your diet. Just as a poor diet and other risk factors can turn your fat genes on, you can turn them back off by filling your plate with the ZERO BELLY foods.

The ZERO BELLY eating plan—you'll find a full list of ingredients, all readily available, on page 88—leverages this new research to maximize your intake of gene-disarming nutrients at every meal. Lean meats, leafy greens, red fruits, dark chocolate, peanut butter, and other ZERO BELLY foods act directly on your fat genes, dampening these actions while quelling the inflammation that can switch them back on. These nutrients are like delicious little IT geniuses, hacking into your body's computer system and shutting off all the switches that have gone haywire, resetting your genetic code to "slim."

ZERO DIABETES

Having diabetes is a lot like being in the middle of the ocean and dying of thirst. You're surrounded by something your body desperately needs, but ingesting it will kill you.

With diabetes, that toxic substance is sugar. Sugar—derived from the various healthy fruits and vegetables we eat—is what our bodies run on; we can't function without it. But when you suffer from diabetes, that very same substance can wreak havoc.

Your digestive system turns brunch into glucose—the form of sugar your body uses for energy—and sends it into the bloodstream. Zap! You got energy. But glucose is actually toxic when it lingers in the bloodstream, so when the glucose hits, your pancreas—a large gland located near your stomach—produces insulin, a hormone, and sends that into the bloodstream as well. Insulin is your body's air traffic controller: it takes command of all your glucose and directs it into your cells, where it can be used for rebuilding muscle, for keeping your heart pumping and your brain thinking, for exercising or singing or dancing, or for doing whatever it is that Miley Cyrus does.

But overeating on a consistent basis—or taking in too many calories too quickly, like when we eat sweets or drink sweetened beverages—turns insulin into the boy who cried wolf. Eventually your body's insulin receptors—the docking stations where insulin parks glucose—begin to ignore insulin's instructions. That's a condition known as insulin resistance. After several years, the pancreas gets fed up with producing all that ineffective insulin and begins to produce less than you need. This is called type 2, or adult-onset, diabetes. (Given that poor diet is the major risk factor, it's no surprise that 80 percent of people with type 2 diabetes are overweight.) Glucose builds up in the blood, turning toxic and damaging the blood vessels, which is why diabetes can result in blindness, impotence, amputation, and other horrible afflictions. But remember, the body needs that glucose, which is now overflowing from the bloodstream and passing out through the urine. So at the same time too much sugar is killing you, you don't have enough sugar in your cells to keep your body functioning. You feel fatigue and unusual thirst, and you begin losing weight for no apparent reason. You get sick more often, and injuries are slow to heal, because your body is losing its ability to maintain itself.

More than 8 percent of the American population has diabetes, and more than a third of us have elevated blood sugar levels. Which should have all of us pissed off, because diabetes is a highly preventable disease. Several studies indicate that belly fat is strongly correlated with risk factors such as insulin resistance, which sets the stage for type 2 diabetes.

Reducing belly fat via exercise and a healthy diet are the two best ways to prevent and manage the disease—and that's just what this book is intended to teach you to do. So adopt the principles of ZERO BELLY, and while you're at it, consider a few additional steps.

CUT YOUR RISK 33 PERCENT

DISCOVER SOMETHING FISHY

There's a reason why omega-3 fatty acids are one of the core ZERO BELLY nutrients. Considered "essential" because the body does not produce them naturally, omega-3s boast a number of health benefits, including helping to reduce the risk of type 2 diabetes. A study by the University of Eastern Finland found that men with the highest intake of omega-3 fatty acids had a 33 percent reduced risk for this type of diabetes, compared to men with the lowest intake. Oily fish like wild salmon, rainbow trout, sardines, and mackerel are among the best sources of omega-3s. The American Heart Association recommends eating two 3 1/2-ounce servings of fatty fish per week.

CIRCUIT TRAIN YOUR BELLY AWAY

Aerobic exercise is known to prevent type 2 diabetes, and combining a heart-pumping cardio session with muscle-strengthening exercises is even better. A study published in the journal *PLOS Medicine* found that women who engaged in at least 150 minutes per week (about 20 minutes per day) of aerobic activity and at least 60 minutes per week (three 20-minute sessions) of muscle-strengthening activities reduced their risk of diabetes by 33 percent compared with inactive women.

GET YOUR GREEK ON

A Mediterranean diet may help to guard against obesity and consequently reduce your risk of diabetes by up to 21 percent, according to research presented at the American College of Cardiology's 63rd Annual Scientific Session. The researchers' conclusion comes from the analysis of nineteen original research studies that followed more than 162,000 participants for an average of five and a half years. While there is no set Mediterranean diet, it commonly emphasizes fresh fruits and vegetables, beans, nuts, fish, olive oil and even a regular glass of red wine—which is exactly where you'll be if you're eating the ZERO BELLY foods.

HIT THE TRAIL MIX

A study at the University of North Carolina at Chapel Hill found that people who consumed the most magnesium from foods and from vitamin supplements (200 mg per 1,000 calories of food intake) were about half as likely to develop diabetes over the next twenty years as people who took in the least magnesium (100 mg per 1,000 calories). Large clinical trials testing the effects of magnesium on diabetes risk are needed to determine whether a causal relationship truly exists, but researchers have found that as magnesium intake rose, levels of several markers of inflammation decreased, as did resistance to the effects of the key blood-sugar-regulating hormone insulin. Higher blood levels of magnesium also were linked to a lower degree of insulin resistance. Pumpkin seeds and dark chocolate are two of the best food sources of magnesium.

EAT THE WHOLE THING

Simply choose a whole apple instead of a glass of apple juice, and not only will you dodge a ton of added sugar and additives, but you may also lower your risk for diabetes, according to a study by the Harvard School of Public Health. Researchers found that people who ate at least two servings each week of certain whole fruits—particularly blueberries, grapes, and apples—reduced their risk for type 2 diabetes by as much as 23 percent in comparison to those who ate less than one serving per month. Conversely, those who consumed one or more servings of fruit juice each day increased their risk of developing type 2 diabetes by as much as 21 percent. Swapping three glasses of juice a week with three servings of whole fruit was associated with a 7 percent risk reduction! The high glycemic index of fruit juice—which passes through the digestive system more rapidly than fiber-rich fruit—may explain the results.

DROP ACID

A study of more than sixty thousand women found that an acid-promoting diet, one that includes more animal products and processed foods than fruits and vegetables, causes a number of metabolic problems including a reduction in insulin sensitivity. According to the study, women with an "acid load" in the top quartile had a 56 percent increased risk of developing type 2 diabetes compared with the bottom quartile. Foods that promote an alkaline body environment—vegetables, fruits, and tea—counter acidity.

GIVE RED MEAT THE RED LIGHT

Bad news for people who love going back for seconds at the barbecue: researchers at the University of Singapore found that a small increase in red meat (we're talking half a serving per day) was associated with a 48 percent elevated risk for type 2 diabetes over the course of four years. The good news is that you can undo some of the damage by reducing your red meat intake.

CHAPTER THREE

WIN THE BATTLE INSIDE YOUR BELLY

How Balancing Your Digestive System in Just Three Days Can Take You from Fat to Flat

I **'ve got some disturbing news for you.**

After consulting with a number of high-level international black-ops contacts—people on the inside at the CIA, the State Department, MI6, Blackwater, and the guy in charge of bailing Justin Bieber out of jail—I've uncovered a shocking truth about your belly.

It's bugged.

In fact, your belly is so heavily bugged that there are about a hundred times as many bugs—single-cell bacteria—in your digestive tract as there are human cells in your entire body. On a per capita basis, you're about 99 percent microbe. In a true democracy, your body would cancel your Match.com account and reproduce only through binary fission.

Fortunately, human cells are much, much bigger than bacteria cells, which is why you look like you and not like a protozoan. But what's happening in your gut does impact your shape in more ways than you might imagine. Indeed, if your midsection is looking more amoeba-like than you'd prefer, one of the reasons may lie deep inside your gut. Before you can reset your metabolism and turn off your fat genes, you need to balance your belly.

THE GOOD, THE BAD, AND THE BUGGLY

The human GI tract contains more than five hundred species of bacteria—trillions of microbes that help to break down food, while also playing a role in knocking off any invading bugs that might be taking a ride on your radicchio. In fact, some of the bacteria in your gut even help ward off the pathogens that cause colds and flus. Think of them as a little miniature battalion of Navy SEALs swimming around below your belly button, doing a lot of the dirty work while remaining always ready to engage in battle on your behalf.

But like any efficient military, your bug brigade needs solid leadership—otherwise, you get chaos and mutiny. A balanced gut means your squirming little squadron is working with maximum efficiency on your behalf. But when things get out of whack—because of a poor diet or, sometimes, medications like antibiotics and even heartburn remedies—the forces below your navel can turn on you.

In fact, the inside of your gut is sort of like *Game of Thrones*, with good families and wicked ones fighting it out for supremacy. (Even the names of the microbe families sound straight from George R. R. Martin: studies show that obese people have higher levels of bad bacteria from the phylum Firmicutes, while lean people have higher levels of good bacteria from the phylum Bacteroidetes.)

Why do you gain weight when your bacteria are out of whack? Well, some of the bacteria in your gut release toxins, which inflame the GI tract. As long as these bacteria are kept in check, that's not a problem. But when they begin to overwhelm the better-trained bacteria, you've got a midsection mutiny on your hands.

As those toxins begin to cause inflammation in your digestive tract—a condition known as "leaky gut"—the complications can be massive. Essentially, think of your intestinal tract as a fine screen, with little tiny holes through which nutrients can move into the bloodstream from your food. When bacteria get out of whack, they begin to irritate the lining of the intestines, and those holes become larger. Bacteria, food particles, and other nasty things escape your GI tract and get into your bloodstream. These pathogens begin to attack the body and the body fights back. The results: inflammation, weight gain, bloating, and fat genes that rev into the red.

On the other hand, when you start to cut out the sugars, preservatives, unhealthy fats, and bloating foods, replace them with ZERO BELLY foods, and allow your gut to begin to heal, you'll start to see real changes.

You'll lose weight. Inflammation caused by an imbalance in your gut can turn on your fat genes, leading you to gain more weight than someone eating the same amount of food, and spending the same amount of time in the gym. (That's why ZERO BELLY places such a premium on restoring your gut health.) In a study published in the *British Journal of Nutrition* in late 2013, researchers looked at overweight men and women who were put on a calorie-restrictive diet and given either a placebo or a probiotic supplement—basically, Navy SEALs reinforcements—for twelve weeks. At the end of the twelve weeks, women who had received the healthy gut bacteria showed significantly greater weight loss than those who had the placebo. Even more impressive, the treatment was then stopped and the subjects measured again twelve weeks later. Those women who got the probiotics kept losing weight, even after stopping treatment, while those who got the placebos started gaining weight back. (Researchers note that the same effect wasn't observed in the male subjects, however.) In another study, adults with "large visceral fat areas" who drank 7 ounces of liquids laced with probiotics lost up to 9 percent visceral fat and 3 percent belly fat, while the control group lost nothing.

Your belly will shrink—rapidly—making you look slimmer in just days. Ever notice how some days you wake up, glance in the mirror, and just look and feel slimmer? And some days you go to button your pants and think, "What happened?" It could be in your head: maybe you're not feeling as fit and fired-up as you normally might be. But maybe it's because you still weigh the same, but you actually do appear fatter thanks to belly bloat— the side effect of an imbalanced gut. According to the American Society for Clinical Nutrition, a healthy bug called *L. plantarum*, a bacterial strain found in plant-based foods, can decrease bloating, particularly in people with irritable bowel syndrome. It's found in the highest concentrations in fermented plant foods like sauerkraut and brined olives.

Your body will start creating the fatty acids that shut down your fat genes. Chronic inflammation caused by a leaky gut is one of the most common culprits for the triggering of fat-storage mechanisms and genes connected to metabolic disorders like insulin resistance. In fact, it's the fatty acid butyrate, produced by healthy bacteria feasting on fiber, that helps to dampen the behavior of genes linked directly to insulin resistance and inflammation. More healthy fiber from the ZERO BELLY foods means healthier bacteria, which means more butyrate and an end to inflammation and diabetes.

You'll get more nutrition from your food, helping you to trim down quickly. Because the microbes in your gut help you pull nutrients out of your meals, any disruption in the sensitive balance within your gut means that less of what you eat winds up being used for fuel—another factor in weight gain.

You'll slash your risk for chronic disease. Inflammation plays a role in asthma, allergies, skin disorders, arthritis, Alzheimer's, heart disease, cancer, and even diabetes. A recent study in the journal *Diabetes* found that the gut microbiota of children with type 1 diabetes (an inherited disease) differ from those of children who don't have the disease. Researchers believe that diet and other external factors may be able to counteract the negative autoimmune effects of an unhealthy gut.

You'll catch fewer colds and flus. Researchers from the Institute of Food Research and the University of East Anglia have discovered that gut bacteria produce an enzyme that modifies how the cells in the lining of your digestive tract communicate. This communication system not only helps your body digest food but also plays a major role in fighting infection.

You'll be less anxious and more happy. And not just because you're spending less money on new pants. Studies now indicate that gut bacteria may play a huge role in our emotional health as well—one reason why GI-related issues like irritable bowel syndrome are usually related to depression or anxiety disorders. Researchers in Ireland found that mice treated with *Lactobacillus rhamnosus*, a gut-healthy bacteria found in dairy products, especially yogurts and hard cheeses, suffered less stress, anxiety, and depression-related behavior.

For just these reasons, it's clear that no diet plan can ignore the role of gut health in fighting inflammation and weight gain. ZERO BELLY is one of the first major diet programs to consider gut health as a significant part of its overall weight-loss strategy. And getting your belly under control is easier than you'd think.

DO NOT FEED THE ANIMALS

You understand how cavities come about, right? When you eat sugary foods, that sugar sticks to your teeth. Bacteria in your

INSTANT BELLY BLOATERS

Some foods and drinks can make you feel like a python that's just swallowed a pig. If you're feeling suddenly gassy and bloated, here are some possible perpetrators of your prodigious protrusion.

CHEWING GUM
CULPRIT: SORBITOL

Chewing gum may seem like a harmless habit, but one too many sticks can give whole new meaning to the phrase "bubble butt." Sugarless gums typically contain sorbitol, a sugar alcohol known for causing bloating and other gastrointestinal distress. Sorbitol takes a relatively long time to digest, and undigested sorbitol in your small intestine acts as a hothouse for the fermentation of bacteria, causing boating and flatulence.

NUTRITION BARS
CULPRIT: SOY PROTEIN

You probably don't think of beans when you unwrap a protein bar, but a lot of them include protein isolate derived from soybeans—something many people find just as gas-

mouth digest the sugar, and that process causes damage to the tooth enamel, which leads to cavities. Brush your teeth often, floss, and eat less sugar, and presto—fewer cavities.

Well, imagine that your belly works the same way. Bad bacteria in your gut feed off sugar, just like the bacteria in your mouth. And a Harvard study recently found that a diet based primarily on animal protein—especially one that involves lots of food pack-

inducing as the musical fruit. Like other beans, soy contains oligosaccharides, sugar molecules that the body can't break down entirely. With nowhere to go, these oligosaccharides hang out in the digestive tract, where they ferment, causing gas and bloating of the stomach.

SOME BRANDS OF ALMOND MILK
CULPRIT: CARRAGEENAN

Almond milk is a better option than cow's milk for those with lactose sensitivity, which is why I recommend it as a great base for ZERO BELLY drinks. But you may be undermining your goals if you're buying a brand with the thickening agent carrageenan. Derived from seaweed, carrageenan has been linked to ulcers, inflammation, and other gastrointestinal problems. If you notice bloating after drinking almond milk, consider switching brands. Trader Joe's, Whole Foods 365, and Westsoy make versions without carrageenan.

DRIED FRUIT
CULPRIT: FRUCTOSE

Nature's candy, dried fruit can be a great source of nutrients and fiber. But it can also be a source of gas for those who suffer from fructose malabsorption, which occurs when the body has difficulty absorbing the natural sugar. Dried fruits are particularly high in fructose; fresh stone fruits, citrus fruits, and berries are safer options for those with sensitivity.

CANNED SOUP
CULPRIT: SALT

Good for the soul but potentially bad for the stomach, soup can hide sky-high sodium counts that may lead to water retention and temporary weight gain. When you overload your system with salt, your kidneys can't keep up; salt that would otherwise be flushed away has to sit in your bloodstream, where it attracts water, causing increased blood pressure and bloating.

aging and burger wrappers—can quickly alter the delicate balance of microbes in your belly as well. Even a short-term change in the balance between animal products and plant products can cause rapid changes in your belly.

That's why ZERO BELLY is low in sugar and so heavily tilted toward plant-based foods. I want you to continue to enjoy steak, eggs, and even bacon, but by cutting down on animal products in the early part of the day, you'll create a hospitable environment for beneficial belly bacteria to blossom. And while you already know that cutting down on sugar means you'll lose weight, you probably had no idea that it would change your whole digestive ecosystem and help prevent a microbial mutiny.

ZERO BELLY BACTERIA RULES

DON'T be fooled by yogurt. To reduce both natural and added sugars, I've cut yogurt out of the ZERO BELLY plan. While yogurt has a reputation for being good for belly bacteria, most yogurts are so high in added sugars that they'll do more for the bad bacteria in your belly than they will for the good. If you do choose to eat yogurt, look for the words "live active cultures" on the label.

DON'T mistake frozen yogurt for a health food. All of the processing that frozen yogurt goes through kills off most of the healthy bacteria.

DO be smart about probiotics. Studies show they have far fewer of the healthy bacteria than they claim. In a Consumer Lab.com study, Nature Made Digestive Health Probiotics, Culturelle, and Align Probiotics all scored high marks. But an adult supplement should have 10 to 20 billion colony-forming units (CFUs) to be effective, far more than what the typical supplement has.

But there's an added ZERO BELLY bonus. While you're cutting down on the sugars and animal proteins that feed the bad bugs, the foods in your new diet will help you pack your day with nutrients that feed the good bugs. In one Canadian study, subjects who were supplemented with a natural insoluble fiber called oligofructose not only lost weight but reported less hunger than those who received a placebo. Researchers discovered that the subjects who received the fiber had higher levels of ghrelin—a hormone that controls hunger—and lower levels of blood sugar. (Oligofructose is found in foods like onions and leeks; oatmeal, rye, and barley; and Jerusalem artichokes.) The reason insoluble fiber works so well in balancing the gut is that it's not digested; it

DO store probiotic supplements in a cool, dry, dark place to avoid damage from heat, humidity, and light.

DON'T try baby poo sausage. Spanish scientists, having discovered that the bacteria in probiotics are also found in abundance in baby poo, have cultured these bacteria and are using them to ferment sausage. But, I mean, really . . .

DO become an astronaut. The Japanese Aerospace Exploration Agency is giving probiotics to astronauts on the International Space Station to see if rebalancing gut bacteria will help reverse health problems caused by zero gravity, such as muscular atrophy and a decline in immune function.

DON'T move to Siberia or Antarctica. Human obesity is associated with having high levels of bacteria from the phylum Firmicutes and low levels of bacteria from another phylum, Bacteroidetes. In a study of 1,020 healthy people from twenty-three countries, researchers found that the further from the equator you live, the more of the bad microbes you are likely to have, and the fewer of the belly-slimming ones.

remains in your GI tract all the way to the end, reaching the good bacteria in the lower intestines and helping them to fight off the bad guys.

The ZERO BELLY menus are also high in omega-3 fatty acids, which help to reduce inflammation, and low in gluten (the protein found in wheat). Recent studies have found that gluten can negatively impact gut bacteria, even in people who are not gluten sensitive.

After reading all of this about belly bugs, you might be wondering: "How come I'm not eating yogurt all day long, or popping those probiotic supplements? Isn't that how you get those healthy gut bugs into your system?"

Well, yes. It's true that some yogurts contain beneficial bacteria that can send reinforcements into the gut when you need them. *Lactobacillus acidophilus* is the bacteria you want to look for, with yogurts that say "live active cultures." But most yogurts are so high in sugar that they do more to promote unhealthy gut bacteria than anything else, which is why I don't recommend them on the ZERO BELLY plan. And while probiotics may help, these supplements are unregulated, and it's not clear whether they pack enough bacterial cultures to make a difference. Consumer Lab.com did a recent study in which its testers looked at twelve popular brands of probiotic supplements and found that they contained far less of the healthy colony-forming units (CFUs) than they claimed. Supplements aren't regulated by the FDA, so there's no way to know whether what's claimed on their labels is accurate when they're shipped out of the factory; worse, though, is that heat, humidity, and time eventually kill off the bacteria, so when it finally gets to you, a probiotic supplement may have few if any living cultures.

But relying on supplements and even yogurt to replenish an unhealthy gut isn't a great idea. It's like stocking fish in a polluted pond. The new fish will eventually die, and then you'll have to ship in more fish. Wouldn't you rather have a healthy pond where the natural aquatic life can live healthfully and thrive forever?

FIFTY SHADES OF FAT

Brown fat, white fat; good fat, bad fat—sometimes it seems like the doctor who understands fat the best is Dr. Seuss. In the past few years, researchers have discovered that, like khakis at the Gap, fat comes in many different shades—each with unique molecular properties and health implications. What does the fat rainbow mean for you? Here's everything you need to know about different body fat types.

BROWN FAT: GOOD FAT

From an evolutionary perspective, brown fat helps to keep a newborn's core temperature warm—it's the brown adipose tissue (BAT) found in the back of the neck, and serves to convert food to heat. It acts like a muscle when stimulated by cold environments, burning calories for fuel. An adult of normal or below-normal weight naturally stores about 2 to 3 ounces of brown fat—enough to burn 250 calories over the course of three hours when stimulated. As for standing in a cold shower to lose weight, theoretically it could work, but the clinical proof of "shivering yourself skinny" has yet to be seen.

BEIGE FAT: GOOD FAT

The neutral-colored fat, identified just two years ago, has been harder to study because it's mixed in with brown and white fat and occurs in tiny pea-size deposits near the collarbone and along the spine. At least in mice, it shows huge potential for weight management. According to the Dana-Farber Cancer Institute, when mice exercise, they release the hormone irsin from their muscles, which converts white fat into brown fat—a process called "browning." Since humans have the same hormone in their blood, researchers suspect humans also produce beige fat via exercise. This fat stores the energy that would otherwise wind up in your belly. Researchers from the University of Texas Health Center at San Antonio found that when stimulated by cold, the body produces a protein called Grb10, which serves as the on-off switch for a molecular pathway that signals white fat cells to turn into brown fat cells. Because the brown and white cells are mixed together, the resulting fat is "beige."

SUBCUTANEOUS WHITE FAT:
NEUTRAL FAT

Dubbed "the inch you can pinch," this kind of white fat—called subcutaneous fat—lies directly under the skin. It's the fat that's measured using skinfold calipers to estimate body fat percentage, and it's found all over the body. While excess fat is never a good thing, subcutaneous fat, particularly around the hips and thighs, is not particularly dangerous. In fact, a study published in the *New England Journal of Medicine* in 2004 found that liposuction removal of subcutaneous fat (up to 23 pounds of it) in fifteen obese women had no effect after three months on their measures of blood pressure,

blood sugar, or cholesterol. So while a muffin top might not be on your list of fashion do's, it's not high on the list of health don'ts. (And as I pointed out earlier, some research indicates that subcutaneous fat may even protect against the onset of diabetes.)

VISCERAL WHITE FAT:
BAD FAT

Visceral fat, often referred to as "deep fat," is energy-storing white fat that wraps around the inner organs. For this reason it's very hard to remove surgically and incredibly dangerous. One reason excess visceral fat is so harmful is that its blood flow drains into the liver via the portal vein. In other words, all the toxins and fatty acids given off by visceral fat are swept up by the blood and dumped into the liver, negatively impacting the production of blood lipids (cholesterol). Research published in the journal *Diabetes* also suggests that visceral fat pumps out immune system chemicals called cytokines that can increase the risk of cardiovascular disease by promoting insulin resistance and chronic inflammation. Abdominal obesity is a state of chronic visceral inflammation. The good news is that because of its rich blood flow, visceral fat is very responsive to exercise—far more so than stubborn subcutaneous fat.

ZERO HEART DISEASE

Clench your fist. Squeeze it a few times. Now imagine that fist inside your chest, pumping over and over, hard enough to pump blood and oxygen throughout your entire body—about sixty thousand miles' worth of veins and arteries—and never resting, 24 hours a day, 7 days a week, 365 days a year.

Is it any wonder your heart needs all the support it can get?

The most important thing your heart needs—besides someone to like your Facebook posts—is a constant, nourishing supply of blood from the coronary arteries. When we talk about heart disease, what we're talking about is basically a hiccup in this critical delivery system: blood flow is blocked and cannot get to the heart to feed it.

Heart disease accounts for about 600,000 deaths every year, making it the leading cause of death in the United States. According to the Centers for Disease Control, coronary artery disease, or atherosclerosis, is the most common type of heart disease among Americans. It occurs when plaque (cholesterol) builds up in the walls of the arteries, narrowing the path through which blood can flow.

Left untreated, plaque can build up enough to cause chest pain and shortness of breath—a condition called angina—or it can block the arteries completely, causing a heart attack, which kills part or all of the muscle. Over 720,000 Americans suffer heart attacks each year, according to the CDC.

There are a number of factors that contribute to your heart disease risk, from things you can't control, such as family history and age, to things you can control a bit, including stress level, cholesterol levels, and blood pressure. But there's one major risk factor for heart disease that you can control: visceral fat. The important point is not whether you have excess fat but *where the fat is.* A study published in the *Journal of the American College of Cardiology* found that normal-weight heart patients who have excess abdominal fat are less likely to survive than obese patients whose excess pounds are concentrated in their thighs and buttocks.

That's why I'm so passionate about the ZERO BELLY program. It's not about losing weight—although you'll lose weight, for sure. It's about targeting the fat that matters most. Adopt the principles of ZERO BELLY, and—especially if you have an elevated risk of heart disease—consider the following heart-specific recommendations.

EAT LESS RED MEAT

Reducing your intake of red meat to just a few times a month, or cutting it out completely, could improve your heart health by altering your gut bacteria. A new study suggests vegetarians and vegans digest meat differently than carnivores, which makes them less susceptible to heart disease. Researchers call it "revenge of the cow," and it starts with L-carnitine—a chemical found in red meat that, when a meat-eater's gut microbes get hold of it, produces a compound called trimethylamine N-oxide, or TMAO, that hardens arteries. But your risk goes up only if you've made a habit of feeding these carnivorous gut bacteria. In studies, longtime vegetarians' microbes didn't produce much TMAO at all when they ate red meat. Additionally, red meat is typically high in saturated fat and cholesterol—two things you want to cut down on when eating for a healthy heart.

EAT 2 SQUARES

. . . Of dark chocolate, that is. Researchers at Louisiana State University discovered that bacteria in our stomach ferment chocolate into useful anti-inflammatory compounds that are good for the heart. Gut microbes such as bifidobacteria feast on the chocolate and release beneficial polyphenolic compounds. The scientists believe that adding fruit to chocolate could boost the fermentation. Chocolate-covered strawberries, anyone?

BREAK UP WITH YOUR SWEET-HEART

Health officials are now pointing the finger at sugar as the leading dietary cause of cardiovascular issues. According to a recent study published in *JAMA Internal Medicine,* the risk of dying from cardiovascular disease more than doubled for those who consumed 21 percent or more of their calories from added sugar. (To put that into frightening perspective: the average American man eats 2,200 calories a day and gets 496 calories, or 22.5 percent, from sugar. The average American woman eats 1,858 calories and gets 400 calories, or 21.5 percent, from sugar.) One of the easiest ways to reduce your added sugar intake is to follow the ZERO BELLY protocol, which cuts out sugary drinks and reduces processed foods—that's anything with a label that lists more than two or three ingredients. But don't worry: you'll still satisfy your sweet tooth with fresh fruits, delicious smoothies and oatmeal bowls, and plenty of delicious desserts.

GET FIT(TER)

Studies suggest a combination of cardio and resistance training is the best fitness formula for the heart. That's what makes ZERO BELLY's metabolic circuits, which combine both aerobic exercise and resistance training, so effective. According to research presented at the American Heart Association's Quality of Care and Outcomes Research Scientific Sessions, middle-aged people who increase their fitness level can radically reduce their risk for cardiovascular issues. For example, if a 40-year-old went from jogging a mile in twelve minutes to running a mile in ten minutes, he or she could reduce risk of heart failure at a later age by 40 percent!

SWAP SALT FOR SPICE

Dietary salt is known to increase blood pressure, which is itself a major risk factor for heart disease. But a directive like "eat less salt" is hard to follow, especially when the nachos are calling your name. The trick: find salt-free ways to bolster the flavor of your food. Adults who participated in a recent twenty-week behavioral intervention that taught them to swap salt for herbs and spices consumed 966 mg less sodium per day than people who tried to reduce sodium on their own. Better yet, certain herbs and spices have proven ZERO BELLY benefits, like boosting the metabolism and blocking fat cell formation. See page 86 for a list of my favorites.

LET IT SPROUT

Ever find gnarly old heads of garlic with green sprouts growing out of them in the bottom of your fridge? Don't toss them! Scientists report that this over-the-hill garlic has even more heart-healthy antioxidant activity than the fresher stuff. Aged garlic extract, also known as kyolic garlic or AGE, has the same effect. A recent study found that participants who took four pills of AGE a day saw a reduction in plaque buildup in the arteries. And the good news is that you don't have to down old garlic; you can find AGE supplements at most drug and health food stores, and it's odorless. (Let the kissing continue!)

FILL UP ON FIBER

Fiber protects the heart by boosting the body's ability to produce low-density lipoprotein (LDL) receptors, which act like bouncers, pulling "bad" cholesterol out of the blood. Researchers at the University of Leeds analyzed a number of studies and found that risk of cardiovascular disease was significantly lower for every 7 grams of fiber consumed—that's just one portion of whole grains, beans, or legumes, or two servings of fresh produce.

GO WILD FOR BLUEBERRIES

Researchers at the University of Maine have revealed wild blueberries as the world's best-tasting aspirin—a natural supplement for cardiovascular health, particularly blood flow to and from the heart. According to their study, wild blueberry consumption (2 cups per day) for eight weeks was shown to regulate and improve the balance between relaxing and constricting factors in the vascular wall in obese rats. Two cups is a lot, but you can up your intake by throwing 1/2 to 1 cup of the blue gems in your ZERO BELLY drinks and your morning oatmeal. Blueberries are surprisingly tasty on green salads too! (Note: You can find wild blueberries in the freezer section of most major supermarkets.)

CHAPTER FOUR

HOW REAL IS YOUR RISK?

The New Gold Standard for Measuring Your Belly Fat Risk, and the Perfect Plan for Beating the Odds

n the previous chapters, I explained some weird science about fat:

• The fat just under your skin (subcutaneous fat) may be ugly, but it's relatively harmless and may even have some benefits.

• The fat buried in your belly (visceral fat) sends out toxic substances that ruin your health and erode your muscular strength.

- Fat comes in different colors, including brown, beige, and white, and each type plays a different role in your body's functioning.

- Fat is approximately 47 percent Republican, 45 percent Democratic, and 8 percent independent.

Okay, that last one was just to make sure you were paying attention.

The exact function of fat cells is one of the long-standing mysteries of biology that science is just beginning to unlock. But what we do know is that fat is a lot more complicated than we once thought. And if different types of fat gather in different places, perform different functions, and either work for you or against you—and if certain kinds of fat actually reduce the size, strength, and quality (and therefore the weight) of your muscles—then it stands to reason that simply standing on a bathroom scale isn't a particularly good measure of how healthy you're becoming.

Indeed, in just the past couple of years, the way that scientists look at the connection between fat, weight, and health has completely changed. The good news: we now have a much better way of telling just how healthy—or unhealthy—we all are.

HOW TO ZERO IN ON YOUR BELLY

For decades, the gold standard in assessing the relationship between health and weight has been a measurement known as the body mass index, or BMI.

While BMI really became popular in the early 1990s, it actually dates from about 150 years earlier. To calculate your BMI, simply divide your weight in kilograms by the square of your height in meters. While that means a bit of annoying metric conversion, it's pretty simple. People whose BMI is between 18.5 and 25 fall in the normal range, while those with a BMI above 25 are considered overweight and those above 30 obese.

Here's a quick way to calculate your BMI. Let's say you're a 5'11" man who weighs 206 pounds. First, multiply your weight by 703.

$$206 \times 703 = 144{,}818$$

Next, calculate your height in inches squared. A 5'11" man is 71 inches. To square that number, times it by itself.

$$71 \times 71 = 5{,}041$$

Now we divide the first number by the second.

$$144{,}818 \div 5{,}041 = 28.7$$

That's not the healthiest number, according to the way BMI is currently assessed.

Problem is, BMI was invented in early 1800s Belgium, using early 1800s Belgians. These were not folks who did a lot of weight training, and there weren't many distance runners, volleyball players, or other folks of unique physical dimensions. So BMI doesn't do a great job of taking into consideration the amazing diversity of Americans' shapes and sizes and fitness levels.

As a result, a 5'11" man who weighs 206 pounds has a BMI of about 28.7, meaning he's considered not just overweight but actually bordering on "obese." But because muscle weighs more than fat, and because fat comes in different forms and is distributed in different ways, that BMI measurement doesn't tell us whether that man is a couch potato or 2014 Super Bowl–winning quarterback Russell Wilson of the Seattle Seahawks, whose body clocks

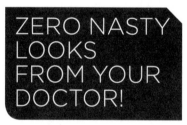

ZERO NASTY LOOKS FROM YOUR DOCTOR!

I saw results immediately. My doctor even congratulated me on my weight loss!

—MARTHA CHESLER, 52,
who lost 21 pounds

in with exactly that BMI, according to his NFL.com stats. And as much of a bummer as BMI might be for the fit and fabulous, it's even more of a problem for those who actually are at risk for illness because of their body mass.

In fact, there's something that's even more dangerous than being too skinny or too fat, according to your BMI: being "skinny fat"—a combination of too much visceral fat and too little muscle. (And remember—visceral fat destroys muscle, so the more visceral fat you gain, the more muscle you lose.)

That's why BMI alone isn't an effective tool for measuring whether or not you're healthy or even overweight. A recent study of 650,000 people, published in *Mayo Clinic Proceedings*, examined the effect of waist circumference on health. The study looked at people with a variety of BMI measurements, including those who fell squarely in the normal range. According to the researchers, those with a higher waist circumference—regardless of BMI—were at greater risk for heart disease, cancer, respiratory problems, and premature death.

In fact, in animal studies, researchers have been able to show that they could increase visceral fat—and, as a result, also increase insulin resistance, total cholesterol, and LDL and triglyceride levels—without increasing body weight. Same BMI and same weight, but a much higher risk of death.

In other words, when it comes to battling obesity with BMI, we've pretty much brought a knife to a gunfight. Fortunately, there's a new weapon in town.

USE YOUR BRAIN TO BEAT YOUR BELLY

Recent studies suggest a new obesity measure called A Body Shape Index, or ABSI, can reveal more about your risk of death and disease than body weight or BMI ever could.

That's because while it takes those numbers into consideration, ABSI also factors in the critical, missing component: waist circumference. In other words, it reveals the truth about your belly fat. If weight and BMI measure "bigness," then ABSI measures "roundness"—and whether your belly puts you at risk.

The ABSI formula was discovered in 2012 by Nir Krakauer, assistant professor of civil engineering in City College of New

A TALE OF TWO BELLIES

Meet Bill and Jack, two regular dudes going about their lives. They started off at college in the same place—but followed their bellies down two very different paths.

1984

Jack and Bill are college buddies who, by coincidence, the same measurements: They're both the average height for an American man, about 5'9"; each weighs 164 pounds, and has a 34-inch waist. Both carry the same health risk as the average 21-year-old American male; their Relative Risk from ABSI is exactly 1.0.

But let's see what happens to Jack and Bill after graduation.

45"

42"

40"

35"

34"

JACK BILL

1984

2004

At their twenty-year reunion, they've both put on a little weight—but so has the rest of the Class of 1984.

Jack, for one, is a bit heavier—but just a bit. At 180 pounds, he's still sporting a 35-inch waist. As a result, Jack's risk of dying is nearly 10 percent lower than that of the average man his age. Most important, the high-nutrient diet that Jack eats has kept his genetic propensity for weight gain in low neutral—his fat-storage genes haven't been tripped. Even though he's gained weight, it's been muscle and a little subcutaneous fat—not visceral fat. As a result, his

Relative Risk calculates at 0.7. He's 30 percent less at risk than the average 41-year-old.

But two decades of working at a desk, exercising irregularly, and eating the typical American diet has pushed Bill's weight up to 192 pounds and his waist is now at 42 inches; the AHA considers him "abdominally obese." (Men with a waist of 40 inches or more and women with a waist of 35 inches or more are considered to have abdominal obesity.) Although their weight isn't dramatically different, their body composition is. A greater percentage of Jack's weight comes from lean muscle tissue; Bill's comes from visceral fat. As a result, his Relative Risk is now 1.7—or 70 percent higher than it should be.

York's School of Engineering, and his father, Jesse Krakauer, M.D. The researchers analyzed body measurements and death rates in more than fourteen thousand adults who had participated in two surveys in the 1980s and 1990s. By comparing survey results with death and cancer diagnosis records, they discovered a positive correlation between big bellies and high chances of death. A follow-up study published in February 2014 in the journal *PLOS*

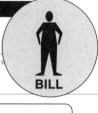

BILL

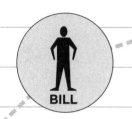

BILL

2024

At their fortieth reunion, both men are 61, and Jack is doing great. By keeping his weight relatively stable, around the 180-pound mark—but more important, keeping his waistline at 35 inches— he's free of metabolic syndrome, and his Relative Risk has stayed the same.

But the decades of bad health decisions have taken a toll on Bill, and his waist is now at a stubborn 45 inches. Despite his efforts to exercise and cut calories,

he can't seem to keep the weight off. "I guess I've got the fat gene," he says. His Relative Risk calculates to 2.1—and Bill is now fully in the clutches of metabolic syndrome. His risk of developing diabetes is six times higher than Jack's. His risk of dying from a heart attack is three times as high. And that belly fat is complicating Bill's life in a lot of ways. Decreased libido, fertility, and erectile function; fatigue, muscle weakness, and headaches; depression, anxiety, and cognitive difficulties—all

have been linked to abdominal obesity.

These aren't imaginary scenarios; they're based on what really happens to average Americans. But it isn't weight gain per se that puts Bill—and the rest of us—at such elevated risk. It's belly fat. And that's what **ZERO BELLY** is designed to help you conquer.

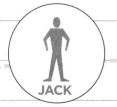

JACK

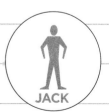

JACK

2004

2024

ONE put a number on that risk: An average ABSI is 1.0. For each 0.1 increase in ABSI, the chance of death increased by 10 percent. People with ABSI in the top 20 percent had death rates 61 percent higher than those in the bottom 20 percent.

To show how this plays out in real life, let's take the example of Katrina Bridges from Bethalto, Illinois. She had tried Atkins, Shakeology, even the Jillian Michaels Body Revolution. Each had helped to a certain extent, but weight was still a battle. Katrina weighed 237 pounds, but the bigger health issue—which she really didn't even know about—wasn't her weight but her waist. Katrina's waist circumference was 50 inches.

Katrina is only 5'5", so her waist size put her in imminent danger. At just 30 years of age, she had an ABSI relative risk of 1.9. What does that mean? Katrina's risk of dying from heart disease or diabetes was 90 percent greater than that of someone with a more modest waist measurement. This mother of three was nearly twice as likely to pass away prematurely.

But after just three days on ZERO BELLY, Katrina noted her stomach had started to shrink. Within just five weeks, Katrina's waist was down to 45 inches, and her ABSI relative risk was down to 1.1. That means her risk of death was just 10 percent greater than that of the average person—an enormous change, and one that can give her children the gift of seeing their mom live a longer, happier life.

To help you quickly figure out your risk, I've put an easy-to-use calculator on www.Zerobelly.com. As you go through the ZERO BELLY program, you'll be able to plug in your numbers and watch as your ABSI—and your risk of diabetes, heart disease, and more—actually shrinks right along with your waist.

First, calculate your waist circumference (WC) by wrapping a measuring tape comfortably around your belly button. (No sucking in—pretend you're being fitted for a new pair of pants that you want to be secure but comfortable.) Then plug in your height and weight, and calculate.

The number to pay attention to is Relative Risk from ABSI, which deviates from an average of 1. For example, if your number is 1.3, you are at 30 percent greater risk of dying from any cause than the average person your age; a number of 0.8 would mean you are at 20 percent lower risk.

However, if you'd like to crunch the numbers yourself—or if you're trapped in a snow cave in the Arctic and the Wi-Fi is a little iffy—you can do it without accessing the Internet by using a formula developed by the Krakauers. You multiply ⅔ of your BMI by ½ your height in inches. Then you measure your waist circumference, and divide that measurement by the earlier number. It's not as confusing as it sounds. Let's stick with Russell Wilson's numbers for an example.

First, multiply your BMI by .66 to find ⅔ of it.

$$28.7 \times .66 = 18.9$$

Now find half your height in inches.

$$71 \times .5 = 35.5$$

Multiply these two numbers.

$$18.9 \times 35.5 = 671$$

Got it so far? Now, apply a tape measure to your waist. Since the folks at *Men's Fitness* put Wilson on the cover of their October 2013 "Game Changers" issue, and shot him without pads, it's easy to estimate that Wilson has a 34-inch waist. So if we divide that number by our calculation, we whould get Wilson's ABSI.

$$34 \div 671 = 0.5$$

The lower that number, the better, but anything over 1.0 is troublesome. An ABSI in excess of 2.0, for example, indicates your risk of dying early is more than double that of the average person.

So while the old measurement, BMI, tells us that Wilson is

bordering on obese, his ABSI says he's actually at a lower risk of dying than the average man. (Although in fairness, ABSI does not take into account blitzing 49ers linebackers.) That's good news for the Seahawks—and even better news for those of us who care about living longer, healthier, and happier.

TIME TO TARGET THE REAL ENEMY

What these numbers, and many other studies, demonstrate is that people with large waists die sooner than those with flat bellies, even if their body weight is normal. The deep abdominal fat wrapped around our internal organs directly increases the risk of diabetes, stroke, and cardiovascular disease.

But there's another way to look at it: Russell Wilson is an all-star both in the NFL and in the ABSI because he has a lot of muscle and very little visceral fat. It stands to reason, then, that losing weight doesn't really matter; losing belly fat is what counts. The most dangerous thing you can have is not fat, not high body weight, but a terrible combination of increased visceral fat and decreased muscle mass.

Fortunately, that's exactly the problem ZERO BELLY was created to fix.

ZERO ALZHEIMER'S

It's a scourge that can turn a bright mind into mush, strip intelligent people of their ability to reason, and reduce bold personalities into frightened shells. No, I'm not talking about cable news channels—although if someone has a cure for Wolf Blitzer, I'm all ears. I'm talking about Alzheimer's, a disease that touches just about all of us at some point in our lives, and one that must be stomped out.

More than five million Americans are estimated to have Alzheimer's disease—a number that's expected to nearly triple by 2050 if there are no significant medical breakthroughs, according to the Alzheimer's Association. Alzheimer's is the most common cause of dementia, a term describing a set of symptoms that can include loss of memory, mood changes, and problems with communication and reasoning. It worsens with time, and it's irreversible. In most people living with Alzheimer's, symptoms first appear after age sixty. The time from diagnosis to death varies—as little as three or four years if the person is older than 80 when diagnosed to as long as ten or more years if the person is younger, according to the National Institute on Aging.

During the course of the disease, protein plaques and tangles develop in the structure of the brain, leading to the death of brain cells. Before long, the damage spreads to a part of the brain called the hippocampus, which is essential in forming memories. People with Alzheimer's also have a shortage of some important messaging chemicals that are involved with the transmission of signals within the brain. As more neurons die, affected brain regions begin to shrink. By the final stage of Alzheimer's, damage is widespread, and brain tissue has shrunk significantly.

Scientists don't yet fully understand what causes Alzheimer's disease. However, the more they learn, the more they realize that two major factors come into play: genes and lifestyle.

About 15 percent of the general population carries the ApoE4 gene, but 25 to 30 percent of people diagnosed with Alzheimer's have it, according to the National Institute on Aging. The gene variant is just one risk factor for Alzheimer's, but scientists say it seems to be an important one—especially for women. A study published in April 2014 in the *Annals of Neurology* found that the gene had only a minimal effect on men, while in women it nearly doubled the risk of developing Alzheimer's or mild cognitive impairment. Women make up nearly two-thirds of the five million people in the United States diagnosed with Alzheimer's, and researchers think ApoE4 may help explain the disparity.

But simply having the gene for Alzheimer's doesn't mean that gene necessarily will be tripped into action. Just as we've learned a great deal about how we can turn on or turn off the fat storage gene, we're learning more about the epigenetics of Alzheimer's as well.

If Alzheimer's runs in your family, it's especially important to make changes to your lifestyle to minimize your risk. Research has shown that people who smoke, and those who have high blood pressure, high cholesterol levels, or diabetes, are at increased risk of developing Alzheimer's. Belly fat, too, puts middle-aged people at an increased risk. According to researchers at Rush University Medical Center, the protein responsible for metabolizing fat in the liver is the same protein found in the part of the brain that controls memory and learning. People with higher abdominal fat actually have depleted this fat-metabolizing protein, making them 3.6 times as likely to suffer from memory loss and dementia later on in life.

You can help reduce your risk with the diet and exercise protocols of ZERO BELLY, and you can also consider these research-suggested tips.

DON'T PANIC, GO ORGANIC

Here's one more reason to support your local farmers and buy organic produce: researchers say exposure to DDT—

a toxin banned in the United States since 1972 but still used as a pesticide in other countries—may increase the risk and severity of Alzheimer's disease, particularly in those over the age of 60. In a study published in *JAMA Neurology*, Rutgers scientists reported that levels of DDE, the chemical compound left when DDT breaks down, were four times higher in the blood of Alzheimer's disease patients compared to those without the disease. People may be exposed to the toxic pesticide by consuming fruits, vegetables, and grains imported from countries where DDT is still being used and eating fish from contaminated waterways. Just one more reason to buy local and organic!

MAKE MIDLIFE MATTER MOST

If there's one time where diet matters most to preventing your risk of Alzheimer's, midlife is it. A recent doctoral thesis—the first ever to investigate the relationship between a healthy diet in midlife and the risk of developing dementia later on—suggests making the healthiest dietary choices in your 50s may reduce your risk of dementia years later by almost 90 percent! A Mediterranean diet, one rich in vegeta-

bles, berries and fruits, fish, and unsaturated fats from nuts, proved to be particularly beneficial. According to researchers, even those who are genetically susceptible to Alzheimer's can at least delay the onset of the disease by reducing intake of the saturated fat typical of meat and dairy.

LEARN ANOTHER LANGUAGE

A recent study published in the journal *Neurology* shows that speaking a second language may delay the onset of three types of dementia. The study found that people who spoke two languages developed dementia four and a half years later than people who spoke only one language. Speaking more than one language is thought to lead to better development of the areas of the brain that handle executive functions and attention tasks, which may help protect against the onset of dementia.

READ AND REST (BUT NOT TOO MUCH)

Use it or lose it. That seems to be true of proper cognitive function, according to a recent study carried out by a team of researchers in Spain. Their findings show that keeping the brain stimulated, and sleeping just long enough for the mind and body to recoup for another day, is the sweet spot for cognitive development. Sleeping more than eight hours or less than six and a lack of cognitive stimulation such as reading were associated with an increased risk of cognitive impairment by 2.6 times in people over 65, according to the study, published in the journal *Revista de Investigación Clínica*.

MUNCH ON TRAIL MIX

A clinical study suggests that elevating brain magnesium through dietary intake prevents synapse loss and reverses memory decline in aging mice with Alzheimer's disease. The study is the first to show a mechanism for reversing cognitive decline in the advanced stages of Alzheimer's and has exciting implications for humans. You can get your fill of magnesium with a handful of pumpkin seeds and dark chocolate chips (at least 70 percent cacao)—two of the very best dietary sources of the mineral.

FEED YOUR HUNGRY, HUNGRY HIPPOCAMPUS

Did you know your brain shrinks as you age? Most susceptible to atrophy is the hippocampus, a part of the brain responsible for memory and spatial reasoning, and the region first attacked by Alzheimer's disease. But recent studies suggest you can prevent atrophy and delay the onset of cognitive decline by fueling your hippocampus with exercise. Researchers at the University of Maryland School of Public Health studied four groups of healthy older adults ages 65 to 89 who had normal cognitive abilities, tracking them over an eighteen-month period. The groups were classified both for low or high Alzheimer's risk (based on gene expression) and for low or high physical activity levels. Of all four groups studied, only those at high genetic risk for Alzheimer's who did not exercise experienced a decrease in hippocampal volume (3 percent). Those who exercised, even those at high risk for Alzheimer's, maintained the volume of their hippocampus. It's like a biceps pump . . . in your brain!

PART TWO

The
ZERO
BELLY
Diet

CHAPTER FIVE

THE POWER OF THE ZERO BELLY FOODS

The Nine Super Nutrients That Target Belly Fat in Three Ways—and Flatten Your Belly for Good!

've given you an understanding of the ZERO BELLY philosophy and how radically this approach differs from most of what passes for weight-loss science out there. By reducing sugars and saturated fats while also focusing on the foods that help keep your gut healthy, you'll strip away unwanted blubber, turn off your fat genes, stabilize your metabolism, and stop the deadly march of inflammation that's contributing to the national epidemic of weight gain and chronic diseases like diabetes and Alzheimer's.

Now, it's time to get up close and personal with the ZERO BELLY foods themselves. Understanding the power of these nine essential food groups will help keep you focused on losing weight day in and day out, hour by hour, and allow you to see the reduction in your belly as fat, bloating, and inflammation begin to fade while lean, strong muscle takes its place.

Throughout the next few chapters, you'll also meet more of the men and women who have changed their lives with ZERO BELLY. The results—rapid, sustainable weight loss, a reduction in waist size, significant improvements in digestive health, and measurable changes in blood markers and even VO2 max (a measurement of the body's overall endurance)—speak for themselves. Their stories will get you excited about diving into the ZERO BELLY plan.

You'll base your eating plan on the following nine ZERO BELLY food groups, each of which helps to fight inflammation, boost metabolism, and—most important of all—turn off your fat genes and reverse your body's tendency to store fat. The plan is designed to provide protein, fiber, and healthy fats at every meal to help boost metabolism and fight hunger; maximize your levels of micronutrients to shut down your genetic fat-storage mechanisms; and minimize excess sugars, refined carbohydrates, and additives that are known to aggravate the stomach and lead to inflammation and weight gain. The result will be not only fast, easy weight loss but an almost immediate sense of energy, a leaner midsection, and a lighter body. (Your pants will fit better within days.)

While these foods provide a simple guideline for what to eat, I also want you to remember to ask yourself these three questions before each meal or snack:

Where's my protein? Protein is the mighty master of muscle, the ferocious foe of fat, the blitzkrieg bombardier of blubber. Lean meats and eggs, plant-based protein powders, and beans are your primary sources. These foods trigger the "shut-off valve" for genes linked to fatty liver, insulin resistance, and visceral fat gain.

Where's my fiber? Stop thinking in terms of carbs or starches and start thinking in terms of fiber. You'll find fiber in fruits, vegetables, beans, and whole grains like quinoa, oats, and brown rice. Follow the fiber to trip the off switch on genes related to obesity and inflammation.

Where's my healthy fat? The greenest, freshest, most luscious salad in the world isn't as healthy as it could be if you don't add a splash of olive oil to it. The reason: healthy fats help our bodies to process the nutrients in other foods, to slow the pace of digestion—keeping us fuller, longer—and to improve our cholesterol profile and reduce inflammation. Olive oil, avocados, nuts and nut butters, chia seeds and flaxseed, and cold-water seafood are all sources of healthy fats. Some healthy fats have an impact on obesity genes; all will help improve your overall health profile.

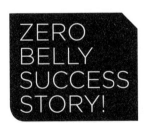

ZERO BELLY SUCCESS STORY!

MATT BRUNNER, 43
Lost 20 pounds and 4 inches in six weeks

"The first week, I lost 7 pounds!"

Despite his fitness-oriented job, 43-year-old Matt Brunner, Director of Athletic Brands at Temple University in Philadelphia, was never able to stay consistent with past weight-loss plans. But he finally found motivation in the rapid results of **ZERO BELLY**. "The first week, I lost 7 pounds!" he says. "It really made me want to keep going." The tasty recipes and clear guidelines helped, too. "The food variety and combinations of MANY different foods made it easy. Plus, the program helped me to understand HOW it works and taught me to adapt meals to stay within the guidelines." The results: "My 'skinny' clothes all look good again!"

I'll explain more about protein, fiber, and healthy fat in the following chapter. But rest assured: If you can look at your plate and find all three, you're having a balanced ZERO BELLY meal or snack. (Even the ZERO BELLY drinks have the right balance to them.)

ZERO BELLY DRINKS
Maximize Nutritional Intake

Each day, you'll enjoy—and I do mean *enjoy*—a blended smoothie designed to complement the natural weight loss and lean muscle gain you'll see from the ZERO BELLY program. These are so delicious, and so simple to make, that you can have them as breakfast, a snack, a meal replacement, or even dessert. Studies show that high-protein, low-fat smoothies are highly effective at rushing nutrients to your muscles—which is why I recommend you have your drink immediately after exercise—and that blended fruit drinks, which include all the fiber, will actually keep you fuller longer than fruit juices.

Perhaps you're thinking, "I already enjoy a protein smoothie. It goes by the name Muscle Milk, or Lean Body, or Met RX, or some other Very Serious Name, and it comes ready to drink! So why do I need these?"

Well, you've already read in earlier chapters how important it is to reduce sugars, saturated fats, and artificial ingredients in order to keep your digestive system properly balanced. And you've seen how an unbalanced gut can cause inflammation, bloating, and weight gain—to the point where having too much of some kinds of belly bacteria puts you at increased risk of obesity.

So why, then, would you drink something that contains carrageenan (a type of seaweed linked to stomach issues); maltodextrin, crystalline fructose, and sucralose (all forms of sugar); cellulose gum and gel (made from chemically digested wood chips); zinc oxide (also used in diaper rash medications); and thirty-six other ingredients—which is exactly what you get when you drink a container of Muscle Milk? Is this helping to foster good gut health? Or does it make you afraid that one night the Toxic Avenger is going to crawl out of your belly button?

By stripping smoothies of the dairy, sugars, and artificial ingredients so common in popular shakes, ZERO BELLY drinks maximize all that's great about protein smoothies while zeroing out the negative. That means you'll be getting optimal nutrition in a delicious, easy-to-digest drink you can have at any point of the day—guaranteed to keep you full, shrink your belly, and leave you feeling full of energy. You'll discover the amazing and delicious recipes starting on page 110.

EGGS
Turn Off Visceral Fat Genes

Eggs are the single best dietary sources of the B vitamin choline, an essential nutrient used in the construction of all the body's cell membranes. Two eggs will give you half your day's worth; only beef liver has more. (And believe me, starting your day with a slab of beef liver does not make for a great morning.)

But as more and more research is done into the mechanisms of our fat genes, the value of eggs has only grown. Choline deficiency is linked directly to the genes that cause visceral fat accumulation, particularly in the liver. (One of the reasons heavy drinkers develop fatty liver is that alcohol undercuts the body's ability to process choline.) Yet according to the 2005 National Health and Nutrition Examination Survey, only a small percentage of all Americans eat daily diets that meet the U.S. Institute of Medicine's Adequate Intake of 425 mg for women and 550 mg for men. Start your day with eggs, and enjoy some other sources like lean beef and seafood.

RED FRUIT
Turn Off Obesity Genes

More and more research has begun to show that some fruits are actually better at fighting belly fat than others. And the master fruits all have one thing in common: they're red, or at least reddish. Check out my favorites:

- **Ruby red grapefruit.** A study in the journal *Metabolism* found that eating half a grapefruit before meals may help reduce visceral fat and lower cholesterol levels. Participants in the six-week study who ate grapefruit with every meal saw their waists shrink by up to an inch. Researchers attribute the effects to a combination of phytochemicals (the more colorful the fruit, the more phytochemicals—which is why ruby red beats white) and vitamin C in the grapefruit.

- **Tart cherries.** Cherries are a delicious, phytonutrient-rich snack. But the true cherry bomb is the tart cherry—not the sort you're used to seeing each summer in bunches at the supermarket. Tart cherries are grown almost exclusively in Michigan, which means that in most of the country you'll find them dried (Whole Foods sells them in bulk), frozen, or canned. But they're worth seeking out because they are a true superpower fruit. A twelve-week study at the University of Michigan found that rats fed tart cherries showed a 9 percent belly fat reduction over rats fed a standard diet. Moreover, researchers noted that the cherries had a profound ability to alter the expression of fat genes.

- **Raspberries, strawberries, blueberries.** They're packed with polyphenols, powerful natural chemicals that can actually stop fat from forming. In a recent Texas Woman's University study, researchers found that feeding mice three daily servings of berries decreased the formation of fat cells by up to 73 percent. Another study at the University of Michigan found that rats who had blueberry powder mixed into their meals had less abdominal fat at the end of ninety days than those on a berry-free diet. ("Hey, Dave, you said *red* berries!" Yeah, but squeeze a blueberry and what color does it stain your fingers? Red. I rest my case.) Blueberries are one of the best sources of resveratrol, the nutrient also found in red wine and red grapes, which has beneficial effects on the epigenetic mechanisms that trigger weight gain and fatty liver.

- **Pink Lady apples.** Apples are one of the very best sources of fiber, which means you should eat them at every opportunity. A recent study at Wake Forest Baptist Medical Center found that for every 10-gram increase in soluble fiber eaten per day, visceral fat was reduced by 3.7 percent over five years. And a study at the University of Western Australia found that the Pink Lady variety had the highest level of antioxidant flavonoids of any apple.

- **Watermelon.** Research at the University of Kentucky showed that eating watermelon may improve lipid profiles and lower fat accumulation. And a study of athletes at Universidad Politécnica de Cartagena in Spain found that watermelon juice helped to reduce muscle soreness—great news if you're following the ZERO BELLY workouts.

- **Plums, peaches, and nectarines.** New studies by Texas AgriLife Research suggest that plums, peaches, and

nectarines may help ward off metabolic syndrome—
a fancy name for the combination of belly fat, high
cholesterol, and insulin resistance. The belly-busting
properties of stone fruits may come from powerful
phenolic compounds that can modulate the expression
of fat genes. (And these fruits also happen to have some
of the lowest amounts of sugar of any fruit.)

OLIVE OIL AND OTHER HEALTHY FATS

Vanquish Hunger

Though it may seem counterintuitive to add fat to a meal if you're
trying to lose fat, eating a moderate portion of unsaturated fats,
like the kind found in olive oil, avocados, and nuts, can ward off
the munchies and keep you full by regulating hunger hormones.
A study published in *Nutrition Journal* found that participants
who ate half a fresh avocado with lunch reported a 40 percent
decreased desire to eat for hours afterward.

And as you may recall from a previous chapter, when
researchers at Uppsala University gave some subjects muffins
made with saturated fat, and others muffins made with polyunsaturated fat, the people eating the muffins made with saturated
fat had gained *primarily belly fat*. This is the first research on
humans to show that the fat composition of your food actually
influences not only your cholesterol levels but also where and
how fat will be stored in your body.

Changing the kind of fat in your diet will also help you
increase your intake of omega-3 fatty acids while reducing

omega-6 fats (found in vegetable oil and fried foods); upping your ratio of omega-3s to omega-6s has been proven to improve metabolic health and reduce inflammation. You'll include a little bit of healthy fat in each of your ZERO BELLY meals.

➜ ZERO BELLY **favorites:** *extra-virgin olive oil, virgin coconut oil, avocados, walnuts, cashews, almonds, almond butter, wild salmon, sardines, ground flaxseed (flax meal), chia seeds.*

BEANS, BROWN RICE, OATS, AND OTHER HEALTHY FIBER
Turn Off Diabetes Genes

Grains get a bad rap because of their carbohydrate content. And now, more and more studies are looking at the effects of gluten, the protein found in wheat, not just as a culprit in weight gain but because of possible long-term health effects like Alzheimer's and heart disease. (In a previous chapter, I mentioned how gluten from wheat can have an adverse affect on gut health, even if you're not gluten-intolerant.) But not all grains are created equal. Gluten-free whole grains like quinoa contain a nutrient called betaine, an amino acid that positively influences the genetic mechanism for insulin resistance and visceral fat.

That's why I want you to stop thinking of "grains" or "carbs" and start thinking of healthy fiber. The right fiber sources provide your body with energy and help to feed lean muscle mass while keeping you full all day. In addition to filling fiber, ZERO BELLY staples like beans, lentils, oats, quinoa, and brown rice contain magnesium and chromium—two incredibly important nutrients that combat cortisol (a stress hormone that directs fat to be stored around the waist) and keep down insulin production (high levels of the hormone also encourage fat to pile on around the belly).

The insoluble fiber found in beans and non-wheat grains help to feed the healthy gut bacteria that improve your chances of staying lean. When the bacteria feed on this fiber, they produce a substance called butyrate, a fatty acid that helps dial down the genes for diabetes and inflammation. You can think of every bean or lentil as the equivalent of a little weight-loss pill. That's not far from the truth. Legumes—foods like beans, peas, and lentils—are

5 FAST MUNCHIE SQUASHERS

You might lose more weight if you exercise an oft-neglected part of your body: your taste buds.

At least, that's what researchers at Deakin University believe. Their new study in the journal *Appetite* suggests that people with a low "taste-threshold for fat" are more likely to overeat due to impaired satiety signals that normally come with a rich meal.

But there's evidence to suggest that healthy eating is a highly sensory experience, and everything from the color of our plates to the sounds in the room may trigger a mindless binge. Here are five ways you can avoid overeating:

Dine by candlelight.
Taking the time to set the mood may increase your meal satisfaction, making you less likely to overeat. A study of fast-food restaurants published in the journal *Psychological Reports* found that customers who dined in a relaxed environment with dimmed lights and mellow music ate 175 fewer calories per meal than if they were in a more typical restaurant environment.

rich in resistant starch, which has a very minimal impact on your blood sugar levels because it passes through the body undigested like fiber, feeding the healthy bacteria at the bottom of your digestive tract. One study found that people who ate ¾ cup of beans daily weighed 6.6 pounds less than those who didn't, even though the bean eaters consumed, on average, 199 more calories per day. And legumes are packed with both muscle-building protein and the essential B vitamin folate. Though beans can be a musical fruit for some, canned varieties that have been soaking long enough to break down much of the gas-causing oligosaccharides will give you less trouble. Look for beans that come in cans

Use contrasting plates.

A study in the *Journal of Consumer Research* found that participants who had low contrast between their food and plates—for example, fettuccini Alfredo on a white plate—served themselves 22 percent more pasta than participants who used brightly colored plates.

Chew times 2.

People who double the number of times they chew before they swallow eat 15 percent less food and 112 fewer calories over the course of a meal, according to a study in the *Journal of the Academy of Nutrition and Dietetics.* That adds up to a 300-calorie savings over the course of a day—enough of a deficit to easily lose half a pound a week.

Add some aromatics.

A study in the journal *Flavour* found participants ate significantly less of a dessert that smelled strongly of vanilla than the same dessert with a more mild scent. Adding fresh herbs and spices is an easy way to get the message to our brains that we're being amply fed—and to take it easy at the dinner table.

Unplug.

People who eat while watching TV, listening to music, or reading consume 10 percent more in one sitting than they would otherwise, found a study published in the *American Journal of Clinical Nutrition.* In fact, distracted eaters go on to eat up to 25 percent more total calories over the course of the day. Texting while eating may be as hazardous as texting while driving!

labled "BPA free," which means you'll be reducing your exposure to a chemical that has been linked to weight gain. Trader Joe's and Eden Organic both sell their food in BPA-free cans.

➡ ZERO BELLY **favorites:** *canned black and garbanzo beans; French green lentils; peas; peanuts and peanut butter; old-fashioned oats (not instant); quinoa; brown rice.*

EXTRA PLANT PROTEIN
Boost Metabolism

A decade ago, when I first wrote *The Abs Diet,* I had already become a fan of protein powders, and I recommended them from the start as a way of burning calories and building muscle. But that program centered around whey protein, and as more and more research points out the importance of gut health—and more and more people find themselves struggling with dairy-related digestion issues—I've discovered a much more belly-friendly alternative.

Plant-based protein powders are a low-sugar, high-fiber alternative to popular dairy-based supplements. I guzzled whey shakes for years and was astonished by how much lighter and leaner I felt when switching to a plant-based blend. A study by the University of Tampa that compared plant protein to whey found it to be equally as effective at changing body composition and boosting muscle recovery and growth. But with less sugar and a healthier fat profile, plant-based proteins will also improve your gut health at the same time as they're fueling your muscles. Hemp, rice, and pea proteins are all good options; however, you'll want to ensure you're getting a complete protein with a full amino acid profile, which is why a blend that combines all three is superior.

→ ZERO BELLY **favorites:** *Vega One All-in-One Nutritional Shake; Vega Sport Performance Protein; Sunwarrior Warrior Blend.*

LEAN MEAT AND FISH
Build Muscle and Turn Off Fat-Storage Genes

Protein is kryptonite to belly fat, and the building block of a lean, toned ZERO BELLY. When you eat protein, your body has to expend a lot of calories in digestion—about 25 calories for every 100 calories you eat (compared with only 10 to 15 calories for fats and carbs). Not only that, protein is more filling. A study published in the *American Journal of Clinical Nutrition* showed that a high-protein meal, as opposed to one high in carbs, increases satiety by suppressing the hunger-stimulating hormone ghrelin.

Now, you may be tempted to grab one of those expensive protein bars instead of sitting down to a decent meal. But the effect isn't the same. Not only are you getting a lot of extra sugar and chemicals, but you're not getting the same fat-fighting effects. Studies show that your body burns more calories digesting whole foods than it does digesting processed foods. In addition, lean meats are key sources of choline, a nutrient that helps turn off the genetic triggers that lead to fatty liver—a new epidemic linked to visceral fat—and methionine and vitamin B_{12}, which unplug genes linked to diabetes and weight gain.

→ ZERO BELLY **favorites:** *boneless skinless chicken breast, lean ground turkey (94 percent lean), lean beef, lamb, wild salmon, shrimp, scallops, cod, tuna, halibut, orange roughy, freshwater fish like pike and sunfish.*

LEAFY GREENS, GREEN TEA, AND BRIGHTLY COLORED VEGETABLES
Stop Inflammation and Turn Off Fat-Storage Genes

Low-energy-density foods like vegetables are crucial to the ZERO BELLY diet, because they add essential nutrients, filling fiber, and volume to meals, all for relatively few calories. Bright colors signal that the vegetables are rich in polyphenols, micronutrients that help to control diet-induced inflammation. Green tea carries catechins, some of which can "turn off" the genetic triggers for diabetes and obesity. And vegetables, especially the leafy kind, have a very low glycemic load—meaning they fill your body up with nutrients without generating a spike in blood sugar.

Research from the University of Otago found that participants felt happier, calmer, and more positive on days when they consumed fruits and vegetables. And a Vanderbilt University study found that people who consumed three or more servings of fruit and vegetable juice each week were 76 percent less likely to develop signs of Alzheimer's over ten years than those who drank fewer than one serving a week.

The key nutrient in leafy greens is folate, a B vitamin that's been linked to everything from boosting mood to battling cancer. It's also a key that locks down genes linked to insulin resistance and fat-cell formation. "It's the B vitamins that play a big role in epigenetics, especially B_{12} and folate," says Dr. Schalinske of Iowa State.

So, which leafy greens should you focus on? A 2014 study at

William Paterson University ranked vegetables by their nutrient density, based on their levels of seventeen different nutrients, especially folate, that have been linked to improved cardiovascular health. Incredibly, the top sixteen were all leafy greens; red bell peppers came in at number seventeen.

Vegetable	Nutrient Density Score
Watercress	100
Chinese cabbage	91.99
Chard	89.27
Beet greens	87.08
Spinach	86.43
Chicory	73.36
Leaf lettuce	70.73
Parsley	65.59
Romaine lettuce	63.48
Collard greens	62.49
Turnip greens	62.12
Endive	60.44
Chives	54.80
Kale	49.07
Dandelion greens	46.34

What's not on the list, by the way, are white root vegetables such as potatoes, turnips, and parsnips. They're low in phytonutrients and high in starch, so they don't get invited to the ZERO BELLY party. Also not included in this program are vegetable staples like broccoli, cauliflower, cabbage, and Brussels sprouts. These cruciferous vegetables can cause bloating and gassiness, especially when eaten raw. I'm not saying don't eat them if you like, but they shouldn't be staples of your dietary game plan.

➡ ZERO BELLY **favorites:** *watercress, Chinese cabbage, spinach, romaine, kale, chard, carrots, zucchini, red bell peppers, grape tomatoes, mesclun greens, leafy green herbs (parsley, oregano, basil).*

YOUR FAVORITE SPICES AND FLAVORS
Turn Off Genes for Inflammation and Weight Gain

Quick quiz: What's piperine?

☐ A nickname for Kate Middleton's hot sister

☐ A compound found in the sweat of Gladys Knight's backup singers

☐ Something flute players spread on their lips to keep them from getting chapped

☐ A secret superfood that comes from the humblest spice of all

New research has shown that piperine—which is released when the waiter from the fancy restaurant uses that giant pepper grinder in front of your face—has some stunning magical powers. In animal studies, piperine has been shown to fight depression, inflammation, and arthritis and enhance the action of other nutrients. In human studies, it's been demonstrated to improve your ability to get a nice tan while spending less time in the sun. Who knew all that could come from a simple pepper grinder?

From a culinary perspective, the genius has always been in the details. What makes an *Iron Chef* winner isn't his or her ability to carve a duck with a Ginsu knife; it's knowing the magic of herbs and spices, and finding the proper balance for each food.

And spices have long been used as weapons to control sodium in the fight against high blood pressure. A recent behavioral study showed adults how to jazz up meals with herbs and spices instead of salt. As a result, the subjects cut nearly 1,000 mg of sodium a day from their intake—that's more salt than you'll find in five bags of Doritos!

Research is showing that herbs, spices, and flavorings do more than add extra bite to your food and help you reduce salt intake. Yellow mustard seeds have high levels of anti-cancer compounds called glucosinolates; cinnamon has been linked to improved insulin response; compounds in turmeric and horseradish have been shown to impact the behavior of your fat-storage genes; and ginger packs high levels of health-boosting phytonutrients. Bottom line: adding yellow, black, and brown spices to your meals means you're boosting the health benefits across the board, while also calming your tongue's desire for more salt and sugar.

And then there's chocolate. The benefits of dark chocolate keep piling up: mental clarity, lowered blood pressure, decreased appetite. A recent study found that a particular type of antioxidant in cocoa prevented laboratory mice from gaining excess weight and actually lowered their blood sugar levels. And another study at Louisiana State University found that gut microbes in our stomach ferment chocolate and boost our body's production of heart-healthy polyphenolic compounds, including butyrate, a fatty acid that decelerates the behavior of genes linked to insulin resistance and inflammation. (Add fruit to the chocolate to boost fermentation and the release of the compounds.) But make sure you're choosing the right kind of chocolate: Look for a cacao content of 70 percent or above, and stay away from Dutch cocoa, as the Dutching process destroys up to 77 percent of the healthy compounds in chocolate.

➜ ZERO BELLY **favorites:** *yellow mustard, black pepper, turmeric, cinnamon, raw apple cider vinegar, dark chocolate with a cacao content of 70 percent or higher.*

OMEGAS OMG!

Good health depends on a proper balance of omega fatty acids. Too bad your average diet is as balanced as a toddler on a Tilt-A-Whirl.

The science around omega fatty acids is confusing—but eating properly to get the right balance of them is crucial. Omega-3 and 6 fatty acids are "essential fatty acids," meaning that we need them for survival but our bodies don't create them naturally—we can only get them through food. Which has worked just fine for us since Neanderthal times, because nature provides a balance of omega-3s (from meats, seafood, nuts, and leafy greens) and omega-6s (from grains, seeds, and also nuts).

Unfortunately, we no longer forage in the forest. As a result, what we eat isn't anywhere close to what nature intended. Whereas once we ate a ratio of 1:1, by some accounts our intake of omega-6 to omega-3 is now at or above 20:1. Here's why that's bad:

Omega-6 fatty acids are pro-inflammatory. Inflammation is important in moderation: it helps protect our bodies from infection and injury, but in excess it can cause severe damage to our organ systems and contribute to diseases, including obesity, diabetes, and depression. A recent study from the University of South Carolina even found that those with a high intake of omega-6 fatty acids have twice the

TOP OMEGA-3 FOODS (mg omega-3/oz)		TOP OMEGA-6 FOODS (mg omega-6/oz)	
Flaxseed oil	14,925	Safflower oil	20,892
Flaxseeds	6,388	Grapeseed oil	19,485
Chia seeds	4,915	Sunflower oil	18,397
Walnut oil	2,912	Poppyseed oil	17,467
Walnuts	2,542	Vegetable oil	16,163
Dried oregano	1,170	Cottonseed oil	14,421
Alaskan salmon	600	Soybean oil	14,361
Herring	488	Sesame oil	11,565
Whitefish	449	Mayonnaise	11,359
Anchovies	414	Sunflower seeds	11,565
Canned tuna (in water)	266	Margarine	11,359
Oysters	188	Peanut oil	9,136
Yellow mustard	137	Caesar dressing	8,112

risk of becoming depressed as those with a balanced omega-6 to omega-3 ratio. Omega-6 acids are found primarily in oils derived from seeds like sunflower and corn.

Omega-3 fatty acids are the exact opposite. They're anti-inflammatory. Found naturally in foods like fish, seafood, nuts, and leafy greens, omega-3 fatty acids have been proven to aid in cholesterol regulation, arthritis, asthma, ADHD, Alzheimer's disease, and yes, they've been found to lessen the effects of depression.

Since most Americans eat more than 20 times as much omega-6s as omega-3s, many dietary experts recommend aiming for something closer to 10:1. But I believe we can, and should, do better. A recent review of studies in the journal *Biomedicine and Pharmacotherapy* found that a ratio of 4:1 was associated with a 70 percent decrease in total mortality. By eating the ZERO BELLY foods, especially eggs, lean meats, beans, and leafy greens, you'll be achieving—or beating—this ratio without even thinking about it. But for extra protection, sprinkle some flaxseeds or chia seeds into smoothies and on salads or oatmeal once in a while, and have a couple of servings of fish a week. That's all it takes to find a perfect balance.

And just as important, be aware of how easy it is to overdose on omega-6s, especially if you like fried foods. The chart on the previous page shows the top sources of 3s and 6s.

Of course, you're probably not meeting friends at the bar for safflower oil shooters. So how do these omega-6 oils make their way into your life? Mostly through fried foods and baked goods, especially from restaurants. Take a look at this list of the biggest downers, based on the highest amounts of omega-6s:

#10. Denny's Fish and Chips:
60,000 mg omega 6
1,330 calories, 73 g fat, 13 g sat fat

#9. Romano's Macaroni Grill Parmesan Crusted Sole:
60,000 mg omega 6
1,550 calories, 104 g fat, 44 g sat fat

#8. IHOP Fried Chicken Dinner:
60,000 mg omega 6
1,570 calories, 84 g fat, 24 g sat fat

#7. Applebee's Chicken Tenders Platter:
66,000 mg omega 6
1,420 calories, 80 g fat, 14 g sat fat

#6. Red Lobster Golden Onion Rings:
75,000 mg omega 6
1,380 calories, 83 g fat, 8 g sat fat

#5. Red Lobster Crispy Calamari and Vegetables:
78,000 mg omega 6
1,390 calories, 88 g fat, 10 g sat fat

#4. Applebee's Hand Battered Fish and Chips:
87,000 mg omega 6
1,560 calories, 105 g fat, 18 g sat fat

#3. Friendly's Kickin' Buffalo Chicken Strips (6 strips):
100,000 mg omega 6
1,650 calories, 116 g fat, 16 g sat fat

#2. Applebee's New England Fish and Chips:
104,000 mg omega 6
1,690 calories, 126 g fat, 22 g sat fat

#1. SADDEST FOOD IN AMERICA Outback Steakhouse Bloomin' Onion:
113,000 mg omega 6
1,959 calories, 161 g fat, 48 g sat fat

SPICE, GIRL!

Recent research has shown that some herbs and flavorings can actually target visceral fat while helping to reduce bloating. Spice rack? That's a fat-fighting utility belt!

GINGER

I cannot confirm whether Confucius had a six-pack, but legend has it the Chinese philosopher ate ginger with every meal. And now there's science to suggest ginger can improve a number of gastrointestinal symptoms. In addition to curing bellyache, a study published in the *Journal of Gastroenterology and Hepatology* suggests ginger may have a unique ability to accelerate gastric emptying. To quote the First Lady: "Let's move!" Freshly grated ginger is delicious in marinades and salad dressings, or pick up a box of ginger tea for a soothing digestif.

BLACK PEPPER

Black pepper has been used for centuries in Eastern medicine to treat multiple health conditions, including inflammation and tummy troubles. And recent animal studies have found that pepper may also have the profound ability to interfere with the formation of new fat cells, resulting in a decrease in waist size, body fat, and cholesterol levels. Season your grilled meats and salads with a few grinds; your waist will thank you.

CINNAMON

Cinnamon contains powerful antioxidants called polyphenols that are proven to alter body composition and improve insulin sensitivity. An animal study published in *Archives of Biochemistry and Biophysics* showed that the addition of dietary cinnamon reduced the accumulation of belly fat. And a series of studies published in the *American Journal of Clinical Nutrition* found that adding a heaping teaspoon of cinnamon to a starchy meal may help stabilize blood sugar and ward off insulin spikes. Sprinkle cinnamon in your morning oats and smoothies for a smaller waist, fewer cravings, and appetite control.

CORIANDER

You can think of coriander as a tastier, less expensive version of Pepto-Bismol. Derived from cilantro seeds, coriander contains a unique blend of oils (specifically, linalool and geranyl acetate) that work like over-the-counter meds to relax digestive muscles and alleviate an overactive gut. A study published in the journal *Digestive Diseases and Science* found that patients with irritable bowel syndrome (IBS) benefited from taking coriander for eight weeks, as opposed to a placebo. Ethnic foods that make good use of coriander can aggravate the tummy, but you can still sneak the spice into marinades, salad dressings, and soups for ZERO BELLY benefits.

MUSTARD SEED

Add mustard to your meal, and feel the burn—literally! Scientists at England's Oxford Polytechnic Institute found that eating 1 teaspoon of prepared mustard (about 5 calories) can boost the metabolism by up to 25 percent for several hours. Not only that, a study published in the *Asian Journal of Clinical Nutrition* found that visceral adipose tissue of rats fed a diet of pure lard was lowered when the diet was supplemented with mustard oil. The ZERO BELLY benefits can be attributed to allyl isothiocyanates, phytochemicals that give the mustard its characteristic flavor. Just be sure you're heating things up with a pure and low-calorie variety (mustard seeds and vinegar). That means avoiding anything that's neon yellow or honey-based.

CAYENNE

A study published in the *American Journal of Clinical Nutrition* found that daily consumption of capsaicin, the chemical that makes cayenne hot, improved abdominal fat loss. And a second study by Canadian researchers found that men who ate spicy appetizers consumed 200 fewer calories at later meals than those who did not. You can find capsaicin in hot sauce, but just a couple of shakes of some popular varieties can provide nearly 20 percent of your daily sodium limit. For a less aggressive, salt-free kick, try seasoning grilled fish, meats, and eggs with just a pinch of cayenne.

THE ZERO BELLY STARTER KIT

This comprehensive inventory of ingredients is all you'll need to unleash the power of the ZERO BELLY foods—to reset your fat genes, reduce bloat and inflammation, fire up your metabolism, and begin losing weight fast, from your belly first. With this handy checklist, you'll have everything you need to create the drinks, snacks, and meals included in this program. These are the healthiest foods on the planet. Feel free to review the recipes, craft your menu, and adjust your shopping list accordingly!

SUPPLEMENT STORE OR ONLINE

Plant-based protein powder blend

Hemp, pea, and rice proteins are all great alternatives to whey. However, a blend is best, as it ensures you're getting a full amino acid profile. As for flavor, vanilla is recommended for most ZERO BELLY drink recipes. Look for a brand with at least 15 g of protein per scoop.

Recommended brands:
- Vega One, All-in-One Nutritional Shake
- Vega Sport, Performance Protein
- Sunwarrior, Warrior Blend

DAIRY

Unsweetened almond milk

Organic eggs

PRODUCE

Apples
(Pink Lady if possible)

Arugula

Asparagus

Avocado

Baby Spinach

Bananas

Bell pepper (red)

Blueberries
(fresh or wild frozen)

Carrots

Celery

Cucumber

Fennel

Garlic

Ginger

Jalapeño pepper

Kale

Lemon

Lettuce
(Romaine, Bibb)

Lime

Mushrooms

Onion (yellow, red)

Raspberries
(fresh or frozen)

Scallions

Strawberries
(fresh or frozen)

Sweet corn

Sweet potatoes

Tomatoes (grape)

Zucchini

CONDIMENTS

Extra-virgin olive oil

Apple cider vinegar

Dijon or spicy mustard
(0 g sugar)

NUTS

Walnuts
(raw, unsalted)

Almonds
(raw, unsalted)

Cashews
(raw, unsalted)

Hazelnuts
(raw, unsalted)

Natural almond butter
(the only ingredients
should be almonds
and salt; Justin's is a
good brand)

Natural peanut butter
(the only ingredients
should be peanuts
and salt; Smucker's
Natural is a good brand)

JARRED AND CANNED

Artichoke hearts

Chipotle peppers

Kalamata olives

Solid white albacore tuna
(packed in water)

Sundried tomatoes

Whole peeled unsalted
tomatoes

PANTRY

Baking soda

Brown sugar

Extra virgin coconut oil

Extra virgin olive oil

Honey

Mirin (sweetened Japanese
rice wine)

Raw apple cider vinegar

Red curry paste

Red wine vinegar

Reduced-sodium
soy sauce

Sake

Sriracha

Unsweetened cocoa
powder

HERBS AND SPICES

Black pepper

Cayenne

Cilantro

Cinnamon

Cumin

Dried bay leaf

Oregano

Rosemary

Salt

Thyme

GRAINS

Long-grain brown rice

Quinoa

Rolled oats (or steel cut)

BEANS & LEGUMES

Black beans

Chickpeas/garbanzo beans

Green lentils

Kidney beans

Pinto beans

PROTEIN

94–99% lean ground
turkey

Chicken breast
(boneless, skinless,
and on the bone)

Halibut

Flank or skirt steak

Shrimp

Smoked Atlantic salmon
(Echo Falls is a good
brand)

Wild salmon

EXTRAS

Salsa (Amy's Organic is a
good brand)

Ground flaxseed
(flax meal)

Dark chocolate, cacao
content 70 percent or
higher (Green & Black's
is a good brand)

Semi-sweet chocolate
chips

Hummus (Abraham's is
a good brand)

Green tea teabags
(Bigelow is a good brand)

Chia seeds

Gluten-free crackers

CHAPTER SIX

THE ZERO BELLY MEAL PLAN

How and When to Eat to Burn Fat and Build Lean Muscle, 24/7/365

Think of the previous chapters as the first half of a superhero movie. You've seen the bad guy and learned of his wicked plot to dominate the world. You've met the good guys, learned about their superpowers, and figured out why they're the best bet for saving the universe.

Now it's time for the battle to begin.

This plan will take all of the information in the previous chapters and boil it down into a simple action plan, one that's going to be easier, more delicious, and more effective than you ever imagined. Here's how to put your weight-loss journey on autopilot.

GUIDELINE 1: FOCUS ON THE BIG THREE

Food can be confusing. I know, because I've been studying health, nutrition, and weight loss for more than two decades, and I still don't know what's in a Slim Jim. (Although in all fairness, most of what's in there isn't actually "food." All I know is that if there were a real truth-in-advertising law, Slim Jim would be renamed Wide Clyde.)

So one of my main goals in writing *Zero Belly Diet* has been to simplify, simplify, simplify, and to make eating healthy as easy as possible. And there may be no simpler way of judging whether a meal or snack is healthy for you than by asking three simple questions:

Where's my protein?

Where's my fiber?

Where's my healthy fat?

Put together a plate that provides all three, and I guarantee you've got a line on a leaner, healthier body that's functioning at the peak of its genetic programming. Hitting all three in one sitting means you're feeding your muscles; eating a slowly absorbed, hunger-controlling meal; maximizing the absorption of nutrients in your food to positively influence your genetics; and striking a major blow against cholesterol and elevated blood sugar. The three macronutrients will also help crowd out refined carbohydrates, saturated fats, added sugars, and other things that I want you to make verboten on the ZERO BELLY plan. Here's the breakdown:

Protein. Protein helps you burn fat in three ways. First, it's the building block of muscle, and you already know that muscle burns fat. Feeding your muscles helps them grow and fight back against the forces of fleshiness. Second, the very act of eating protein actually burns calories. It takes more than a kiss from a princess to turn a frog—or a cow, pig, or chicken, or a nut or a bean, for that matter—into a human. About 25 percent of the calories you eat in the form of protein are burned up just digesting the protein itself (carbs and fat burn up no more than 10 to 15 percent of their calories). And third, protein keeps you fuller longer—in part because that intense digestive process means your body perceives you as being satiated. In a 2013 study published in the journal *Appetite*, women were fed low-, moderate-, or high-protein afternoon snacks. Those who ate the most protein had the lowest levels of hunger and waited longer before they chose to eat again than those who ate lower-protein snacks.

Fiber. As I mentioned in the previous chapter, I want you to stop thinking about "good carbs" or "bad carbs" and start focusing on fiber. If you're eating fiber, you're eating nuts and seeds, fruits and vegetables, beans and other legumes, and whole grains. That means you're packing your day with foods high in folate, vitamin B_{12}, betaine, resveratrol, and sulforaphane—all critical nutrients that impact how active our fat-storage genes are. Fiber also allows the bacteria in your gut to produce the fatty acid butyrate, which influences the behavior of genes associated with insulin resistance and inflammation.

Fiber plays a number of additional roles in keeping us slim, but the most intriguing is its ability to suppress appetite. In spring 2014, an international team of researchers identified an anti-appetite molecule called acetate that's naturally released when fiber is digested. Acetate then travels to the brain, where it signals us to stop eating.

Some scientists believe that the dramatic reduction in fiber in our diets is perhaps the number-one factor in our obesity crisis. Professor Gary Frost from the Department of Medicine at Imperial College in London, who was part of the team that put together the acetate study, estimates that, thanks to food processing, the average Western citizen now eats about one-seventh as much fiber as humans did in the Stone Age. Makes you want to chew through a redwood, doesn't it?

Healthy fat. I'm not here to be a goaltender for your mouth every time you try to put a Whopper in it. But I do want you to understand that a fast-food burger, fries, and a shake have plenty of fat, none of it healthy. If you want a ZERO BELLY meal or snack, it needs to contain at least one of the following ingredients:

Monounsaturated fats: olives and olive oil; nuts (including peanuts) and nut butters; avocado; dark chocolate (at least 72 percent cacao)

Polyunsaturated fats: oily fish such as tuna, salmon, mackerel, or sardines; flaxseed; sunflower seeds; sesame seeds; pine nuts

Plant-based saturated fats: coconut (no sugar added), coconut oil (not hydrogenated)

Omega-3 fatty acids: wild salmon, tuna, sardines, and other cold-water fish; grass-fed beef; flaxseed; walnuts; chia seeds

Though it may seem counterintuitive to add fat to a meal if you're trying to lose it, eating a moderate portion of unsaturated fats, like the kind found in olive oil, avocados, and nuts, can ward off the munchies and keep you full by regulating hunger hormones. As I mentioned earlier, studies show that those who eat monounsaturated fats like avocado at lunchtime report a decreased desire to eat for hours afterward. Moreover, increasing the amount of omega-3 fatty acids in your diet while reducing omega-6 fats (found in vegetable oil and foods fried in that oil) has been proven to improve metabolic health and reduce inflammation.

Pop quiz: If you've been paying attention, you've noticed that there's one simple food that, eaten in isolation, gives you all of the Big Three in one simple, bite-size package. Nuts are high in fiber, protein, and healthy fats, and popping a handful into your tank means you're in ZERO BELLY territory from the first bite. Peanuts work too; they're good sources of genistein and resveratrol, powerful anti-obesity gene hackers. Skip commercial trail mixes and canned nut mixes, which are often coated with oil, sugar, and salt, and buy nuts raw and in bulk to save money and calories. When you're buying peanut butter or other nut butters, check the ingredients list: there should be no mention of sugar, oil, or any other additives. Peanuts and maybe a little salt, that's it; if there's anything on the label besides that, pick another brand.

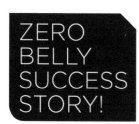

BRYAN WILSON, 29
Lost 19 pounds and 6 inches in six weeks

"ZERO BELLY allows you to indulge and lose weight without grumbling through the pain of diet restriction!"

A 29-year-old accountant, Bryan was happy with his career and success. But when it came to his health, there was room for improvement. At 316 pounds with a bloated 46-inch waist and little idea as to what sustainable—and satiating—healthy eating looked like, Kyle was at a loss. He'd tried other diets, like Weight Watchers, but tired of the point counting and severe calorie restriction that left him feeling hungry and defeated. ZERO BELLY was just the thing for Bryan. "The program actually allows you to eat good food. Almost immediately I lost the bloat"—a result Bryan attributes to the high-protein, dairy-free ZERO BELLY drinks. "I love them. I'm a sweets craver, and these were an awesome alternative to the bowls and bowls of ice cream I would have had."

GUIDELINE 2: EAT THREE MEALS AND ONE SNACK A DAY

If you want to look leaner and feel better, you need to keep your metabolism burning hot. And that means providing your system with the right fuel—often. On the ZERO BELLY plan you'll be eating up to five times a day, including three square meals, at least one ZERO BELLY drink, and one afternoon or evening snack (if you're still hungry). There's science to support the fact that eating more meals works at keeping your metabolism roaring, but the plain-speak reason it works is because it does something that many diets don't do: it keeps you full and satiated, which will reduce the likelihood of a diet-destroying binge or too-large meal that can leave you bloated and uncomfortable.

Below are two possible eating schedules. If you're planning on following the ZERO BELLY workouts, and typically exercise during the day, enjoy a ZERO BELLY drink as a mid-morning snack, to provide you with the extra energy you need to power through a workout. If you choose to exercise at night, or on days when you won't be exercising, enjoy your drink in the afternoon. A study published in the *Journal of the American Dietetic Association* found that mid-morning snackers were more likely to graze mindlessly throughout the day, resulting in more daily calories and a compromised weight-loss effort. In contrast, afternoon snacking was associated with a slightly higher intake of fiber, fruits, and vegetables.

SAMPLE SCHEDULE: LUNCHTIME WORKOUT

7:30 a.m.	Breakfast
10:00 a.m.	ZERO BELLY Drink
12:00 p.m.	Workout
1:00 p.m.	Lunch
6:30 p.m.	Dinner
7:30 p.m.	Snack or ZERO BELLY Drink (optional)

SAMPLE SCHEDULE: NO WORKOUT

7:30 a.m.	Breakfast
12:00 p.m.	Lunch
3:30 p.m.	Snack or ZERO BELLY Drink
6:30 p.m.	Dinner
7:30 p.m.	Snack or ZERO BELLY Drink (optional)

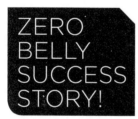

ZERO BELLY SUCCESS STORY!

BOB McMICKEN, *51*
*Lost 24 pounds and
6 inches in six weeks*

"Before ZERO BELLY *I felt bloated and depressed. I finally feel flat. And I'm smiling!"*

A hardworking food service director and father of seven, Bob McMicken knows stress. And at 229 pounds with a dangerously large waistline, he knew his health was a major concern. Sick of feeling bloated and emotionally drained, Bob made a commitment to taking control of his health and signed up for **ZERO BELLY**. Within days of following the easy menu, Bob's bloat seemed to disappear. And in less than six weeks, Bob had lost 24 pounds and a whopping 6 inches from his formerly distended middle. "Before **ZERO BELLY** I felt bloated, fat, and depressed," he said. "Now I feel better, have more energy, and am smiling! I found my favorite shirt finally covered my belly again!"

GUIDELINE 3: HAVE ONE ZERO BELLY DRINK EACH DAY

One of the goals of ZERO BELLY is to maximize the amount of fat-burning, muscle-building, inflammation-fighting, gene-hacking nutrition that goes into your body every day. And the truth is, there's already a lot of food in this program. So I've made it super easy to pack in even more weight-loss magic in the form of the ZERO BELLY drinks.

These smoothies solve a lot of problems. First, they're so delicious and easy to make you can have them for breakfast, for a snack, or even for dessert. Second, they ensure that you'll stay satiated and satisfied all day long. In a study presented at the North American Association of the Study of Obesity, research-ers found that regularly drinking meal replacements increased a person's chance of losing weight and keeping it off longer than a year.

GUIDELINE 4: PREP SOME POWER FOODS FOR ZERO STRESS

At the beginning of each week you'll prep a few essential ZERO BELLY ingredients in bulk, including frozen bananas for your smoothies and brown rice and quinoa for your meals. Lentils may also be prepared in advance, depending on how often you choose to include them in your meal plan. (Vegetables and drinks should be prepared at time of serving to prevent oxidation and maintain optimal nutrition.) The overall goal here is to eliminate that moment when you walk into the kitchen and think, "Hmmm, what should I eat?" which inevitably leads to dialing Domino's. By prepping dinner in advance, you'll never wonder what to eat: It's already made for you!

ZERO STRESS PREP RECIPES

BROWN RICE

Slow-release carbs like brown rice and quinoa beat weight gain and diabetes in three ways: they're top sources of the nutrient betaine, which helps dampen the action of genes related to insulin resistance; they're packed with fiber that helps produce butyrate, a fatty acid that turns off genes related to inflammation and insulin resistance; and they provide long-lasting energy without the blood-sugar spikes associated with other carb-rich foods.

I've found the easiest way to prepare brown rice in bulk is to boil it like pasta for half the recommended cooking time and then steam it till tender.

Prep for 8 servings (about 4 cups total)

- 1 **cup long-grain brown rice**
- 8 **cups cold water**
- 1 ½ **teaspoons salt**

• Rinse the rice with cold water for 30 seconds. Drain.

• Bring the water and salt to a boil over high heat in a large, heavy pot with a tight-fitting lid. When the water is boiling, add the rice, stir, and partially cover (don't cover completely or it will spill over) and cook on medium-high heat, like pasta, for 30 minutes.

• Drain the rice in a strainer, then quickly return to the pot and cover tightly for 20 minutes so the steam finishes cooking the rice.

QUINOA

Quinoa is a complete protein with a full amino acid profile. It's light and fluffy in texture but has that whole-grain ability to fill you up, and the same gene-hacking powers as brown rice.

>   1 **cup quinoa**
>   2 **cups cold water**
>   ½ **teaspoon salt**

• Rinse quinoa under cold water for 30 seconds. Drain and transfer to a medium pot.

• Add water and salt and bring to a boil.

• Cover, reduce heat to medium-low, and simmer until water is absorbed, 15 to 20 minutes.

• Set aside off the heat for 5 minutes. Uncover and fluff with a fork.

GREEN LENTILS

Lentils are a ZERO BELLY favorite. A half-cup serving delivers 3.4 grams of resistant starch, a healthy carb that resists full digestion and boosts metabolism. Cooked lentils will keep refrigerated for about a week.

Quick tip: Any amount of lentils can be cooked in this manner. Just maintain a 2:1 ratio of water to lentils

>   1 **cup dried green lentils**
>   2 **cups water**
>   1 **bay leaf, garlic clove, or other seasoning**
>   ¼–¾ **teaspoon salt**

• Rinse dried lentils in a colander and transfer to a saucepan. Cover with the water and the bay leaf and any seasonings. Reserve the salt. Bring the water to a rapid simmer over medium-high heat, then reduce the heat to maintain a very gentle simmer. Cook, uncovered, for 20–30 minutes. Add water as needed to make sure the lentils are just barely covered. Lentils are cooked as soon as they are tender and no longer crunch. Strain the lentils and remove the bay leaf or garlic clove. Return the lentils to the pan and stir in salt.

ZERO BELLY VINAIGRETTE

There's developing research to suggest vinegar can aid weight loss by keeping our blood sugar steady. One study among pre-diabetics found the addition of 2 tablespoons of apple cider vinegar to a high-carb meal reduced the subsequent rise in blood sugar by 34 percent. Shake up this recipe in a mason jar and you'll have delicious, additive-free dressing for the week!

Yield: 1 cup, about 16 servings

- ⅓ cup raw apple cider vinegar
- ⅔ cup extra-virgin olive oil
- 1 ½ teaspoons Dijon mustard
- 1 ½ teaspoons honey
- ¼ teaspoon salt
- ¼ teaspoon black pepper

• Combine ingredients in a mason jar and shake vigorously until emulsified.

• Store in fridge and shake before serving.

> Per Tbsp: 83 calories, 9 g fat, 0 g fiber, 0 g protein

FROZEN BANANAS

Not only do frozen bananas provide a luxurious creaminess and natural sweetness to your ZERO BELLY drinks, but studies have shown bananas to positively impact gut health by increasing the good bacteria in our bellies and helping to reduce bloat. Better yet, they're a cinch to prepare. I recommend freezing 10–12 at the beginning of each week.

• Carefully peel the banana so that it stays intact. (Do not make the mistake of freezing the banana with the peel on, which just basically gives your fruit a bullet-proof vest that you won't be able to penetrate.) Discard the peel and cut each banana in half.

• Place up to 12 peeled banana halves into a resealable plastic freezer bag. Remove the air from the bag and seal tightly.

• The bananas will keep in the freezer for a few months. When you're ready to blend, remove the bag from the freezer and grab the amount of bananas needed.

GUIDELINE 5:
GET LEAN WITH ZERO BELLY LIQUIDS

I hate to tell you to drink water, because you've been hearing that advice since kindergarten. But drinking about eight glasses a day is key to ZERO BELLY results. Not only will the water keep you satiated (a lot of times what we interpret as hunger is really thirst), but water flushes out the waste products your body makes when it breaks down fat for energy or when it processes protein

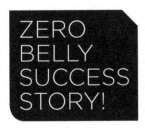

ZERO
BELLY
SUCCESS
STORY!

ISABEL FIOLEK, 55
Lost 13 pounds and 2 inches in six weeks

"One of the regular younger guys at the gym called me skinny—it made my day!"

Isabel wanted a structured program to lose weight fast and get in shape for summer. "I had three weddings to attend—and dresses that were all too small," she said. The six-week ZERO BELLY program was her solution. Once-a-week meal prep and naturally sweet oatmeal and ZERO BELLY drinks were the key to Isabel's success. "I'm toned overall and especially in my midsection. I think I have a two-pack!" More important, she made dramatic health strides: A checkup after her six weeks on ZERO BELLY revealed she'd dropped her total cholesterol by 25 percent and her blood glucose level by 10 percent. And as for those weddings? "I'm now able to fit into my favorite dresses!"

and burns fat. (In other words, the more successful this program is for you, the more water you'll need!) You also need water to transport nutrients to your muscles, to help digest food, and to keep your metabolism clicking.

If you're serious about shedding belly flab, I'd encourage you to cut out booze, soda, and any artificially sweetened drinks for the six-week plan. These drinks are loaded with sugars and artificial ingredients that can cause weight gain and bloating. The easiest way to get in your eight glasses of H_2O is to drink a glass as soon as you wake up, with every meal, ZERO BELLY drink, or snack, and before you go to bed.

You can also have unlimited amounts of green tea, which is rich in catechins, substances that blast adipose tissue by revving the metabolism, increasing the release of fat from fat cells (particularly in the belly), and then speeding up the liver's fat-burning capacity. One particular catechin in green tea, called

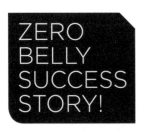

JUNE CARON, 55
Lost 15 pounds and 4 inches in six weeks

"I'm leaner and more energized, and everyone says I look much younger!"

June had tried every diet and exercise program in the book (and on DVD) but grew tired of the repetition and slow results. Frustrated with how menopause had caused her to gain excess weight around her middle (never a problem area before) and determined to get her self-confidence back, a skeptical June decided to give **ZERO BELLY** a shot and dropped 6 pounds within the first week of following the meal plan. "Learning to eat real, chemical-free, fresh foods has been the best thing that ever happened to me. I am never hungry. And the weight just keeps coming off!" Glowing skin, healthy nails, and better sleep were **ZERO BELLY** bonuses, June says. "I'm well on my way to getting my sexy back. Everyone says I look much younger!"

epigallocatechin-3-gallate, has been shown to reduce the activity of genes for obesity, insulin resistance, and fatty liver. In a recent study, participants who combined a daily habit of 4–5 cups of green tea each day with twenty-five minutes of exercise lost 2 more pounds than the non-tea-drinking exercisers! (You'll find a list of my favorite teas for weight loss on page 268.) Meanwhile, a research team in Washington found that roughly the same amount of coffee (5 or more cups per day) doubled visceral belly fat. Limit your coffee to a single cup per day.

GUIDELINE 6:
BREAK THE RULES ONCE A WEEK—WITH ZERO GUILT!

What if I told you that you could cheat, guilt free, and it would actually be good for you? No, not cheating in sports, like Lance Armstrong, or in politics, like Vladimir Putin, or in love, like so many on Capitol Hill. I mean cheating on your diet . . . and reaping some unexpected benefits. In fact, when it comes to weight loss, dietary cheaters almost always prosper. That's because under the right parameters, a weekly "cheat meal" has been proven to boost your metabolism and ward off feelings of deprivation—improving not only your ability to lose weight but your ability to stick to your diet plan as well. One way these meals can boost metabolism is by increasing levels of leptin, the "anti-starvation" hormone responsible for sending hunger messages to the body. When you diet, leptin levels drop, prompting the metabolism to slow down and conserve energy. Throwing a calorie-rich cheat meal into the mix tricks your system into thinking food is plentiful and that it's okay to burn through its fat stores.

Your zero-guilt cheat meal can be anything you want (yes, even pizza), and you can schedule it at any point in the week without derailing your ZERO BELLY results. Note: Don't plan a cheat meal for a big date, because a lot of dieters experience cheat-meal sweats and hot flashes as the metabolism fires up to accommodate the flood of calories.

SAMPLE MEAL PLAN

	Monday	Tuesday	Wednesday
BREAKFAST	Thin Elvis Oatmeal pg. 119	Hash It Out pg. 122	Cherry Pie Oatmeal pg. 119
LUNCH	Keen-Whaaa? Salad pg. 126	Confetti Salad pg. 129	Mediterranean Dinosaur Salad pg. 127
ZB DRINK	Blueberry Dazzler pg. 114	Strawberry Banana pg. 114	Vanilla Milkshake pg. 115
DINNER	Cashew Gesundheit! pg. 135	Halibut à la UPS pg. 136	Quirky Turkey Burger pg. 141
SNACK (OPTIONAL)	Zero Belly Cookies pg. 146	Almond, Brothers pg. 147	Grown-up Goldfish pg. 148

Thursday	Friday	Saturday	Sunday
Simple Frittata pg. 121	PB&J Oatmeal pg. 120	Olé Omelet pg. 123	Blue Ribbon Oatmeal pg. 120
Creature from the Green Legume pg. 128	Hard-Boiled Detective Salad pg. 130	Voodoo Chili pg. 125	Going Lentil Soup pg. 124
The Peanut Butter Cup pg. 115	Mango Muscle-Up pg. 115	Vanilla Milkshake pg. 115	Strawberry Banana pg. 114
Sake-Eye Salmon pg. 134	The Ultimate Burger pg. 140	Chicken of the Mediterranean Sea pg. 131	The M*A*S*H Grill pg. 133
Apple & Nut Butter pg. 147	Zero Belly Cookies pg. 146	Choco- Popcorn pg. 147	Apple & Nut Butter pg. 147

7 HABITS OF HIGHLY SUCCESSFUL LOSERS

There's a surprisingly thin line between loving your body and hating it. Here are some no-diet, no-exercise ways to start losing weight and keeping it off.

1 Lean People Don't Diet

Studies show that the number-one predictor of future weight gain is being on a diet right now. That's primarily because dramatically cutting calories reduces strength, muscle mass, and bone density—and you need strong muscles to burn visceral fat and keep it from recruiting more cells into its fat storage scheme. ZERO BELLY doesn't restrict calories dramatically and always keeps you sated.

2 Lean People Don't Go Fat Free

A European study tracked 90,000 people for several years and discovered that participants who tried to eat "low fat" had the same risk of being overweight as those who ate whatever they wanted. ZERO BELLY is the opposite of low fat; in fact, you'll want to focus on eating healthy fats at every meal.

Lean People Sit Down and Eat

Greek researchers recently reported that eating more slowly and savoring your meal can boost levels of hormones that make you feel fuller. While the ZERO BELLY drinks and snacks are great when you're on the go, the delicious recipes you'll find in this book will make you want to sit down and truly indulge.

Lean People Know What They're Going to Eat Next

Dutch researchers posed a group of test subjects a series of questions like, "If you're hungry at 4:00 p.m., then ... what?" Those who had an answer ("I'll snack on some almonds") were more successful at losing weight than those who didn't. ZERO BELLY sets you up for success by giving you a prep day where you'll stock your fridge with a week's worth of ready-to-eat food, so you'll never have to ask, "What's for dinner?"

Lean People Eat Protein

In recent studies, people who ate moderately high levels of protein were twice as likely to lose weight and keep it off than those who didn't. You'll read more about the magic power of protein in coming chapters, and why protein is part of every single ZERO BELLY meal, snack, and drink.

Lean People Stay Active

While the ZERO BELLY workouts are designed to strip away fat from your belly quickly and effectively, you don't need a formal exercise plan in order to stay lean. You do, however, need to carve out time to move around. The average person makes two hundred decisions every single day that affect his or her weight. Train yourself to say yes to movement.

Lean People Watch Less TV

In a study, participants who cut their daily TV time from five hours a day to two and a half hours a day burned an average of 119 more calories each day. That may not seem like a lot, but over the course of a year, that's enough to lose more than 12 pounds. Over the course of five years, that's a swing of 60 pounds.

CHAPTER SEVEN

THE ZERO BELLY DRINKS

Fat-Melting, Muscle-Building, Gut-Healthy Drinks—Ready in Minutes!

Simple, immediate, and stress free. That's what I want ZERO BELLY to be: a plan that pays off for you quickly, without a lot of hassle and effort. And a key part of that plan is the simple, immediate, and stress-free recipes for ZERO BELLY drinks.

Remember, each time you eat (or drink) a meal or snack, you want to ask three questions:

Where's my protein?

Where's my fiber?

Where's my healthy fat?

ZERO BELLY drinks are plant-based concoctions that are high in all three macronutrients; each of these recipes is perfectly calibrated so the answer to all three questions is "Right here in my glass!" That's the convenience factor: no mind-bending thinking, just blending and drinking.

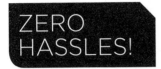

I loved the ZERO BELLY *drinks!*

—ISABEL FIOLEK, *who dropped 13 pounds in six weeks*

The ZERO BELLY test panelists identified the drinks as one of their favorite parts of the program. Bryan Wilson, who lost 19 pounds and 6 inches off his waist, counts the drinks as one of the key components of his success: "I'm a sweets craver and can't get enough ice cream, ever. These were a far better alternative."

The ZERO BELLY drinks are designed to be creamy, filling, and packed with protein, fiber, and healthy fats. But they won't weigh you down with the lactose and saturated fats found in commercial smoothies, most of which rely on dairy-based whey protein and lots of chemicals and preservatives. Cutting out the dairy reduces the bloating and inflammation that can cause your belly to expand.

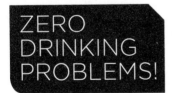

I loved the drinks. They were all pretty easy, and I am sold on protein shakes.

—KATRINA BRIDGES, *who lost 5 inches off her waist*

Because they're plant-based, these smoothies also help ensure that you're getting the nutrients you need to shut off your fat genes—particularly fiber and resveratrol (both found in abundance in red fruits, peanut butter, and dark chocolate)—and reduce the inflammation that can turn them back on. In fact, researchers at Baylor College of Medicine found that dieters who drank 8 ounces of plant-based juices a day over a twelve-week period lost, on average, 4 pounds more than dieters following the exact same plan, but without the drinks.

And the benefits of drinking away inflammation go well beyond just weight loss. A Vanderbilt University study found that people who consume three or more servings of fruit- and vegetable-rich drinks each week are 76 percent less likely to develop Alzheimer's over a ten-year period than those who do not drink them.

Plant-based proteins will also help reduce serum cholesterol and, according to a report in the *American Journal of Clinical Nutrition*, offer "very significant metabolic advantages for the prevention . . . of diabetes." A more recent study in the same journal found that fruit-based drinks could neutralize the inflammatory effects of high-fat, high-carb meals.

Here are a couple of rules to keep in mind as you explore the ZERO BELLY drinks:

• **Freeze!** Don't fall for the common misconception that you need to always use fresh fruit. Beyond being more affordable, the fruit you find in the freezer section is normally picked at the height of the season and flash-frozen. It also makes for colder, creamier smoothies. Simple rule of thumb: If a fruit is at the peak of its season, buy it fresh. If not, stick with frozen. (If you don't use frozen fruit, you can add a cube or two of ice to each recipe.) And don't forget to use the frozen bananas you made at the beginning of the week!

• **Mix up the milks.** Almond and coconut milk are commonly available in most markets, but don't hesitate to experiment with whatever non-dairy milks are on hand at your local market: hazelnut, hemp, rice, and oat milk all can add a creamy dimension to any of these recipes.

One to avoid: soy milk. Soy is particularly high in naturally occurring compounds called estrogenics, which raise estrogen levels and lower testosterone levels, which promotes fat storage. That doesn't mean you need to avoid soy at all costs, but most Americans eat far more soy than they know. I've chosen to leave soy out of ZERO BELLY recipes for just these reasons.

- **Blend like a pro.** Add liquids first, then protein and fruit to your blender. It's easier on the blender and gets things moving faster. For a thicker, spoonable smoothie, use less liquid than dictated by the recipe. Add more for a thinner, milklike consistency.

- **Mess around.** Consider these recipes the base, to which you can add all varieties of nutritional enhancements. Consider turbo-charging your drinks with a handful of baby spinach. The color may change, but the taste change is almost impossible to detect, and it's a great way to get more gene-hacking folate into your day.

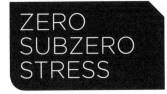

ZERO SUBZERO STRESS

ZERO BELLY *drinks are best right out of the blender, because once you crush up a food, its nutrition starts to deteriorate rapidly. So if you want to take a* ZERO BELLY *drink to travel, consider making it the night before and freezing it in a blender bottle. (Look for one with a metal mixer ball, which helps reblend the drink when you shake it.)*

ZERO BELLY DRINKS

BLUEBERRY DAZZLER

Makes 1 serving

> 1 scoop vegetarian protein powder*
> ½ cup unsweetened nondairy milk
> (almond, hazelnut, coconut, hemp, etc.)
> ½ cup frozen blueberries
> ½ tablespoon almond butter
> Water to blend (optional)

• Combine ingredients in a blender and blend until smooth.

> 232 calories; 6 g fat; 3 g fiber; 28 g protein

* Note: All nutritional stats calculated using Vega Sport Performance Protein (Vanilla). Exact nutritional content may vary based on your choice of plant-based protein powder.

STRAWBERRY BANANA

Makes 1 serving

> 1 scoop vegetarian protein powder
> ⅓ cup frozen strawberries
> ¼ frozen banana
> ½ tablespoon almond butter
> ½ cup unsweetened nondairy milk
> (almond, hazelnut, coconut, hemp, etc.)
> Water to blend (optional)

• Combine ingredients in a blender and blend until smooth.

> 232 calories; 5 g fat; 4 g fiber; 29 g protein

THE PEANUT BUTTER CUP

Makes 1 serving

    1 scoop vegetarian protein powder
  ½ frozen banana
  ½ tablespoon peanut butter
  1 tablespoon unsweetened cocoa powder
  ½ cup unsweetened nondairy milk
     (almond, hazelnut, coconut, hemp, etc.)
     Water to blend (optional)

• Combine ingredients in a blender and blend until smooth.

> 258 calories; 6 g fat; 5 g fiber; 30 g protein

MANGO MUSCLE-UP

Makes 1 serving

    1 scoop vegetarian protein powder
  ⅔ cup frozen mango chunks
  ½ tablespoon almond butter
  ½ cup unsweetened nondairy milk
     (almond, hazelnut, coconut, hemp, etc.)
     Water to blend (optional)

• Combine ingredients in a blender and blend until smooth.

> 224 calories; 5 g fat; 3 g fiber; 29 g protein

VANILLA MILKSHAKE

Makes 1 serving

    1 scoop vegetarian protein powder
  ½ frozen banana
  ½ tablespoon peanut butter
  ½ cup unsweetened nondairy milk
     (almond, hazelnut, coconut, hemp, etc.)
     Water to blend (optional)

• Combine ingredients in a blender and blend until smooth.

> 248 calories; 6 g fat; 3 g fiber; 29 g protein

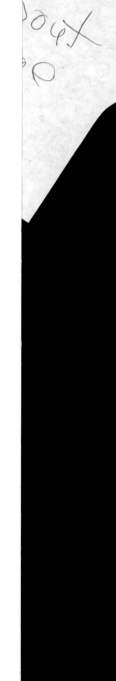

CHAPTER EIGHT

THE ZERO BELLY RECIPES

How to Turn the Zero Belly Foods into Delicious, Easy-to-Make Meals

When **people ask me** what's so unique about the ZERO BELLY meal plan, I tell them this: It involves eating food.

By that I mean real food—food with the power to reverse the fat-gene switches that are triggered by our modern, processed diets and set us back on the path to perfect health.

In 2013, I wrote *Eat It to Beat It*, which looks at the additives in food and how these ingredients are making us fat—by causing inflammation and digestive distress. In fact, studies show that the more processed food you eat, the greater your weight—even if you eat the same number of calories.

Let me repeat that: eating processed foods instead of real

foods will make you gain weight, even if you're eating the same number of calories.

It all goes back to inflammation, and why I built ZERO BELLY to calm the fire and turn off the fat-storage genes that processed foods turn on.

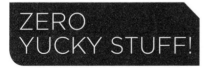

The best thing about the food and nutrition were that they made sense. And let's not forget—they taste great!

—FRED SPARKS, *who dropped 21 pounds and 5 inches off his waist in six weeks*

Today there are more than three thousand food additives approved for use by the Food and Drug Administration. Which is a frightening fact in and of itself, but made worse by the reality that the FDA doesn't actually test these additives for safety. Instead, they rely on food manufacturers to tell them whether or not these chemicals can be "generally recognized as safe." That's how things like wood chips (in shredded cheese and ice cream), plastic foam (in baked goods), duck feathers (in bread), and ingredients from embalming fluid, rocket fuel, and antifreeze wind up in our food.

The ZERO BELLY solution is real food—real, simple food— and easy-to-follow recipes that ensure you're getting the fiber, protein, and healthy fats that will strip away belly fat, fast.

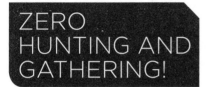

I found all the foods I needed for the plan at my local grocery store, used the plan as a guide, and improvised a menu that worked for me.

—MARTHA CHESLER, *who lost 21 pounds and stripped 7 inches off her waist in just six weeks*

As always, when you're sizing up a potential meal or snack—at home or at your favorite restaurant—ask yourself:

Where's my protein?

Where's my fiber?

Where's my healthy fat?

If you've got all three covered, chances are you're well on your way to ZERO BELLY.

ZERO BELLY BREAKFASTS

One core ZERO BELLY breakfast starts with oatmeal—which you can make using quick-cooking oats every morning or, if you're a more traditional steel-cut type of person, cleverly cook in a big batch earlier in the week, so all you need to do is nuke and go. Starting your day with a bowl of slow-burning oatmeal will help to regulate your hunger and provide your body with powerful beta-glucans, compounds that act like bouncers for low-density lipoprotein (LDL) cholesterol, shuttling that bad cholesterol right out of the VIP room that is your belly. And by pairing your oats with fruits rich in vitamin C, you're going to double the effect—the result of organic compounds called phenols interacting to stabilize cholesterol levels, according to a study published in the journal *Nutrition*.

The second go-to for breakfast is eggs. Eggs are among our best sources of the B vitamin choline and the amino acid methionine, which dampen the activity of genes related to insulin resistance, obesity, and fatty liver disease. They also provide powerful protein punches, which help fire up your metabolism and keep you full throughout the morning rush.

OATMEAL RECIPES

THIN ELVIS

Makes 1 serving

- 1 cup water
- ½ cup quick-cooking oats
- 1 tablespoon peanut butter
- ½ banana, sliced
- Dash cinnamon (optional)

• Bring the water to a boil. Stir in the oats and cook until soft, about 3 minutes. Just before the oats are finished, stir in the peanut butter and banana.

> 302 calories, 10 g fat, 7 g fiber, 10 g protein

CHERRY PIE

Makes 1 serving

- 1 cup water
- ½ cup quick-cooking oats
- 1 tablespoon hazelnuts
- ½ cup dried tart cherries, sliced
- Dash cinnamon (optional)

• Bring the water to a boil. Stir in the oats and cook until soft, about 3 minutes. When the oats are finished, top with hazelnuts and cherries.

> 215 calories, 8 g fat, 8 g fiber, 6 g protein

BLUE RIBBON

Makes 1 serving

- 1 cup water
- ½ cup quick-cooking oats
- ½ cup blueberries
- 1 tablespoon flaked almonds
- Dash cinnamon (optional)

• Bring the water to a boil. Stir in the oats and cook until soft, about 3 minutes. Just before the oats are finished, stir in the blueberries. Top with flaked almonds.

> 251 calories, 8 g fat, 7 g fiber, 8 g protein

PB&J

Makes 1 serving

- 1 cup water
- ½ cup quick-cooking oats
- 1 tablespoon natural peanut butter
- ½ cup strawberries or raspberries

• Bring the water to a boil. Stir in the oats and cook until soft, about 3 minutes. Just before the oats are finished, stir in the peanut butter and berries.

> 269 calories, 11 g fat, 7 g fiber, 9 g protein

PEACHY KEEN

Makes 1 serving

- 1 cup water
- ½ cup quick-cooking oats
- 1 tablespoon flaked almonds
- ½ cup peaches or nectarines, sliced
- Dash cinnamon (optional)

• Bring the water to a boil. Stir in the oats and cook until soft, about 3 minutes. When the oats are finished, top with almonds and fruit slices.

> 220 calories, 7 g fat, 6 g fiber, 8 g protein

EGG RECIPES

SIMPLE FRITTATA

Makes 2 servings (2 wedges per serving)

- ½ tablespoon olive oil
- 1 red bell pepper, sliced thinly
- 1 cup sliced mushrooms
- 1 clove garlic
- 4 cups baby arugula or baby spinach
- 3 whole eggs
- 3 egg whites
- Salt and black pepper to taste
- Herbs and spices to taste

• Preheat the broiler. Heat the oil in a nonstick pan over medium heat. Add the sliced bell pepper, mushrooms, and garlic and sauté until softened. Stir in the arugula and cook for another 2 minutes, until slightly wilted. Meanwhile, whisk together the eggs and egg whites. Put the eggs on top of the vegetables. Season with salt, pepper, and herbs and spices of your choice. Cook on stovetop for 5–6 minutes, until most of the egg has set. Place the pan under the broiler and cook for about 3 minutes, until the rest of the egg has fully set and the top begins to brown. Cool slightly, cut into 4 wedges, and serve.

> 228 calories, 12 g fat, 3 g fiber, 19 g protein

BETTER-THAN GREEN EGGS AND HAM

Makes 1 serving

- 1 large Portobello mushroom cap
- ½ tablespoon olive oil, divided
  Salt and black pepper to taste
- 1 egg
- 2 egg whites
- ⅛ avocado, thinly sliced
  Herbs and spices of your choice

• Preheat the broiler. Line large baking sheet with foil. Remove and discard mushroom stem. Brush both sides of mushroom cap with half the olive oil and sprinkle with salt, then place gill-side up on the baking sheet. Broil mushroom until soft, about 5 minutes per side. Heat the remaining oil in a nonstick pan over a medium-low heat. Whisk the egg and whites in a bowl, add to pan, and scramble. When eggs are just set, remove from heat. Top mushroom cap with eggs and sliced avocado. Season with salt, pepper, and spices of your choosing.

> 226 calories, 14 g fat, 2 g fiber, 17 g protein

HASH IT OUT

Makes 4 servings

- 1 sweet potato, peeled and cut into ¼" cubes
- ½ tablespoon olive oil, divided
- 1 yellow onion, chopped
- 1 red bell pepper, chopped
- ½ cup black beans, drained and rinsed
- ⅛ teaspoon cayenne (optional)
  Salt and black pepper to taste
- 4 eggs

• Microwave cubed potatoes for 5 minutes, or until slightly soft. Heat half the oil in a large nonstick skillet and add the potato, onion, and bell pepper; sauté till they begin to brown, about 7 minutes. Add the beans, along with the cayenne, salt, and pepper, and stir until warmed through. Meanwhile, in a separate skillet, fry the eggs sunny-side up in the remaining oil. Divide the hash among four plates, top with eggs, and serve.

> 187 calories, 8 g fat, 5 g fiber, 10 g protein

OLÉ OMELET

These homemade refried beans keep well in the fridge, so feel free to adapt this recipe for one (that's one whole egg and one egg white) and enjoy a speedy breakfast for the rest of the week!

Makes 4 individual omelets

- 1 can black beans, drained and rinsed
  Juice of one lime
  Dash of hot sauce (optional)
- 4 eggs
- 4 egg whites
  Salt and black pepper to taste
- 4 tablespoons bottled salsa
  (Amy's Organic is a good brand)
- ½ avocado, sliced

• Pulse the black beans, lime juice, and a few shakes of hot sauce (optional) in a food processor until it has the consistency of refried beans. Coat a small nonstick pan with cooking spray and heat over medium heat. Crack one egg and one egg white, combine in a bowl with salt and pepper, whisk, and add to the pan. Use a spatula to stir and lift the cooked egg to let the raw egg slide under. When the eggs have all but set, spoon a quarter of the black bean mixture down the middle of the omelet. Use the spatula to fold over a third of the egg to cover the mixture, then carefully slide the omelet onto a plate using the spatula to flip it over at the last second to form one fully rolled omelet. Top with salsa and avocado. Repeat with the remaining eggs.

> 232 calories, 9 g fat, 6 g fiber, 17 g protein

ZERO BELLY LUNCHES

GOING LENTIL SOUP

Makes 6 servings

- 1 tablespoon olive oil
- 1 medium onion, minced
- 2 cloves garlic, minced
- 1 tablespoon fresh minced ginger
- ½ jalapeño, minced
- 2 medium carrots, peeled and diced
- 1 cup dried green lentils
- ¼ teaspoon cumin
- 1 bay leaf
- 1 can lite coconut milk
- 3 cups low-sodium vegetable stock or water
- 1 tablespoon reduced-sodium soy sauce
- 1 tablespoon red wine vinegar
- Salt and black pepper to taste
- Chopped cilantro for garnish

• Heat olive oil in a medium-size pot set over medium heat. Add onion, garlic, ginger, jalapeño, and carrots and sauté until the onions are soft and translucent, about 3 minutes. Add the lentils, cumin, bay leaf, coconut milk, and stock (or water). Turn heat to low and simmer until the liquid has reduced and the lentils are tender, about 30 minutes. Season with the soy sauce, vinegar, and salt and pepper to taste. If you like, use a hand blender to gently puree the soup for a thicker texture. Garnish with cilantro.

> 300 calories, 12 g fat, 9.5 g fiber, 11 g protein

VOODOO CHILI

Makes 4 servings

- 1 tablespoon olive oil
- 1 medium onion, minced
- 1 medium zucchini, diced
- ½ pound cremini mushrooms, diced
- 1 medium carrot, diced
- 1 red or green bell pepper, diced
- 2 cloves garlic, minced
- 1 can (28 ounces) whole peeled tomatoes
- 2 canned chipotle peppers, finely chopped
- 1 teaspoon chili powder
- ¼ teaspoon ground cumin
- ½ teaspooon dried oregano
- 1 can pinto beans, drained
- Salt and black pepper to taste
- ½ avocado, sliced

• Heat the oil in a large saucepan or pot set over medium heat. Add the onion, zucchini, mushrooms, carrot, bell pepper, and garlic and cook, stirring frequently, until the vegetables are soft and lightly browned, about 10 minutes.

• Add the tomatoes, crushing lightly between your fingers to give the chili a coarse texture. Add the chipotle, chili powder, cumin, oregano, and beans, plus salt and pepper to taste. Turn heat to low and simmer for 20 minutes. Serve in bowls and top with sliced avocado.

> 220 calories, 7 g fat, 9 g protein, 10 g fiber

KEEN-WHAAA? SALAD

Makes 4 servings

> 2 **cups cooked quinoa** (see page 101 for prep recipe)
> **Salt and black pepper to taste**
> 1 **bunch asparagus, woody ends removed**
> 1 **tablespoon olive oil**
> 1 **cup cooked green lentils** (see page 101 for prep recipe)
> ¼ **cup chopped sundried tomatoes**
> ¼ **cup store-bought pesto** (Note: while there is some Parmesan in pesto, the amount in this recipe is unlikely to cause gastrointestinal discomfort. If you run into issues, consider swapping for ¼ cup Zero Belly vinaigrette and a handful of chopped fresh basil instead!)
> 1 **tablespoon Zero Belly Vinaigrette** (see page 102)

• Preheat the oven to 450°F.

• Bring a pot of water to boil, season with salt, and cook the quinoa until just al dente, about 20 minutes. Drain in a colander.

• While the quinoa cooks, drizzle the asparagus with olive oil and season with salt and black pepper. Place in the oven and cook until gently browned and softened, about 10–12 minutes, depending on the thickness of the asparagus. Chop into bite-size pieces.

• In a large mixing bowl, combine the quinoa with the lentils, asparagus, and sundried tomatoes. Mix together the pesto and Zero Belly Vinaigrette, then add it to the bowl of quinoa. Toss to combine.

> 205 calories, 12 g fat, 8 g protein, 6 g fiber

MEDITERRANEAN DINOSAUR SALAD

Makes 1 serving

- 2 **cups chopped kale** (preferably lucinato or dinosaur kale), **ribs removed**
- ¼ **cup cherry tomatoes, halved**
- 4 **Kalamata olives, pitted, halved**
- ¼ **cup artichoke hearts** (canned in water, preferably)
- ¼ **cup cooked chickpeas**
- ⅛ **red onion, diced**
- 1 **tablespoon Zero Belly Vinaigrette** (see page 102)
  Salt and black pepper to taste

• Before making the salad, spend a few minutes massaging and squeezing the kale. It sounds funny, but roughing up the leaves will help break down the tough fibers of the green and make the kale more tender.

• Combine the kale, tomatoes, olives, artichoke hearts, chickpeas, and onion in a mixing bowl. Toss with the vinaigrette and season with salt and black pepper to taste.

> 273 calories, 12 g fat, 10 g protein, 8 g fiber

CREATURE FROM THE GREEN LEGUME

*Test Panel Favorite

Makes 2 servings

- ½ cup dried French green lentils
- 2 large eggs
- ½ cup diced red bell pepper
- 2 tablespoons chopped green onions
- ¼ cup diced celery
- 2 tablespoons Zero Belly Vinaigrette (see page 102)
- 4 cups baby spinach
   Black pepper

• Place lentils in a medium saucepan. Cover with water to 3 inches above lentils; bring to a boil. Reduce heat, and simmer 20 minutes or until lentils are tender. Drain and keep warm.

• Add water to a large saucepan to a depth of 3 inches; bring to a boil. Add eggs; boil 5 minutes and 30 seconds. Drain. Plunge eggs into ice water; let stand 5 minutes. Drain and peel. Eggs will be soft-cooked.

• Toss lentils, bell pepper, onions, and celery in a bowl with 1 tablespoon Zero Belly Vinaigrette.

• Place remaining tablespoon of Zero Belly Vinaigrette and baby spinach in a large bowl; toss to coat.

• Divide spinach between two plates and top with lentils. Cut eggs in half lengthwise; top each serving with 2 egg halves. Sprinkle with pepper and serve.

> 279 calories, 6 g fat, 23 g protein, 9 g fiber

CONFETTI SALAD

*Test Panel Favorite

Makes 2 servings

½ can (5 ounce), solid white albacore tuna,
  water packed (or salmon)
½ cup canned kidney beans
⅓ cup frozen organic super sweet corn
1 cup romaine lettuce, chopped
1 tablespoon Zero Belly Vinaigrette (see page 102)
  Fresh herbs of your choice (optional)

• Break up tuna in bowl; add remaining ingredients and give it
a good mix!

> 304 calories, 11 g fat, 24 g protein, 7 g fiber

HARD-BOILED DETECTIVE SALAD

Makes 2 servings

- 4 cups leafy greens
- ½ cup bell peppers, cut into thin strips
- ½ cup carrots, shredded
- ½ English cucumber, sliced into half-moons
- 2 hard-boiled eggs, quartered
- 2 tablespoons dried tart cherries
  (or sliced fresh berries or grapes)
- 2 tablespoons Zero Belly Vinaigrette (see page 102)

• Combine all ingredients in a bowl and give it a good mix!

> 218 calories, 15 g fat, 10 g protein, 4 g fiber

ZERO BELLY DINNERS

CHICKEN OF THE MEDITERRANEAN SEA

Makes 4 servings

- ¼ cup pitted olives
- 1 tablespoon capers
- ½ tablespoon olive oil
- 10 fresh thyme branches
  (or ½ teaspoon dried thyme or rosemary)
- 2 tablespoons red wine vinegar
- ½ cup white wine
- ½ tablespoon honey
- 4 bone-in, skin-on chicken breasts
  Salt and black pepper to taste
- 4 roma tomatoes, halved
- 4 medium carrots, peeled
- 1 large yellow onion, peeled and quartered

• Combine the olives, capers, olive oil, thyme, vinegar, wine, and honey in a mixing bowl and gently stir. Season the chicken all over with salt and pepper and add to the bowl. Marinate in the refrigerator for at least two hours, but preferably overnight.

• Preheat the oven to 425°F. Spread the tomatoes, carrots, and onion wedges in a roasting pan and season with salt and pepper to taste. Place the chicken breasts on top of the vegetables, then drizzle the marinade all over. Roast in the oven until the chicken is lightly browned and cooked all the way through, about 25 minutes.

> 257 calories, 7 g fat, 27 g protein, 3.5 g fiber

SKINNY THAI

Makes 4 servings

  1 teaspoon coconut oil
  1 medium onion, sliced
  1 medium zucchini, chopped
  4 ounces shitake mushrooms, stemmed and sliced
  1 large carrot, peeled and sliced into ¼-inch rounds
  2 cloves garlic, minced
  1 tablespoon fresh minced ginger
  1 tablespoon red curry paste
  1 can lite coconut milk
  1 pound medium shrimp, peeled and deveined
    Juice of one lime, plus another lime, quartered
    Chopped cilantro for garnish
    Chopped walnuts or peanuts for garnish

• In a large saucepan or pot, heat the oil over medium heat.
Add the onion, zucchini, mushrooms, carrots, garlic, and ginger
and cook until the vegetables are soft and nearly cooked through,
about 7 to 10 minutes.

• Add the red curry paste and continue cooking for 2–3 minutes.
Stir in the coconut milk and turn the heat down to low.
Simmer for 10 minutes. Add the shrimp and cook until they turn
pink and curl gently, about 3 minutes. Stir in the lime juice.

• Divide the curry among four bowls. Serve garnished with cilantro, chopped walnuts, and a lime wedge.

> 218 calories, 11 g fat, 18 g protein, 2.5 g fiber

THE M*A*S*H GRILL

Makes 4 servings

- 1 pound flank or skirt steak
- ¼ cup low-sodium soy sauce
- 1 tablespoon brown sugar
- ½ tablespoon coconut oil
- 3 tablespoons rice wine vinegar
  (white wine vinegar can be substituted)
- 1 English cucumber, thinly sliced
  Salt
- 1 head Bibb lettuce, leaves separated
- 2 cups cooked brown rice
  Sriracha or other Asian chili sauce for serving
  Hoisin for serving

• Combine the steak, soy sauce, brown sugar, coconut oil, and 1 tablespoon of the vinegar in a sealable plastic bag. Marinate in the refrigerator for at least 4 hours and up to 24 hours before cooking.

• An hour before cooking, combine the sliced cucumber with a pinch of salt and remaining vinegar in a small bowl. Set aside.

• Preheat a grill, grill pan, or cast-iron skillet over medium-high heat. Cook the steak 3–4 minutes per side, until a nice crust develops on the surface and the meat is firm but yielding to the touch.

• Serve the steak with the lettuce leaves for wrapping, plus the rice, cucumbers, Sriracha, and Hoisin for topping.

> 320 calories; 8 g fat; 29 g protein; 3 g fiber

SAKE-EYE SALMON

Makes 4 servings

- 4 **4–6 ounce wild salmon fillets**
- ¼ **cup low-sodium soy sauce**
- ¼ **cup mirin** (sweetened Japanese rice wine)
- ¼ **cup sake**
- 1 **bunch asparagus, woody part of the stems removed**
- 1 **teaspoon extra-virgin olive oil**
  Salt and black pepper to taste
  Sesame seeds for garnish

• Combine the salmon, soy sauce, mirin, and sake in a sealable plastic bag. Allow to marinate at least 4 hours and up to 24 hours before cooking.

• Preheat oven to 425°F. Place the salmon in a roasting pan. Toss the asparagus with enough oil to lightly coat, plus salt and pepper to taste, and place them next to the salmon in the pan. Cook the salmon until lightly browned on the outside and the fish flakes with gentle pressure from your finger. Garnish with sesame seeds.

> 247 calories, 7 g fat, 26 g protein, 2.5 g fiber

CASHEW GESUNDHEIT!

*Test Panel Favorite

Makes 4 servings

- ⅓ cup coarsely chopped unsalted cashews
- 2 tablespoons virgin coconut oil
- 1 pound boneless, skinless chicken breast, cut lengthwise into thin strips
- 2 cups julienne-cut red bell pepper (about 1 large)
- 1 teaspoon minced garlic
- ½ teaspoon minced peeled fresh ginger
- 3 tablespoons thinly sliced scallions
- 1 cup cooked brown rice

• Heat a large nonstick skillet over medium-high heat. Add cashews to pan; cook 3 minutes or until lightly toasted, stirring frequently. Remove from pan.

• Add coconut oil to pan, swirling to coat. Add chicken to pan; sauté 2 minutes or until lightly browned. Remove chicken from pan and place in a bowl.

• Add bell pepper to pan; sauté 2 minutes, stirring occasionally. Add garlic and ginger; cook 30 seconds. Return chicken to pan; cook 1 minute. Sprinkle with cashews and scallions. Serve with brown rice.

> 350 calories, 19 g fat, 28 g protein, 2 g fiber

HALIBUT À LA UPS

Makes 4 servings

- 4 **sheets parchment paper** or large pieces of aluminum foil
- 1 **pound halibut** (other firm white fish such as swordfish or mahi mahi will work as well) cut into 4 equal pieces
- 1 **tablespoon olive oil**
  Salt and black pepper to taste
- 4 **thin slices lemon**
- 1 **pint cherry tomatoes**
- 1 **bulb fennel, thinly sliced**
- 8 **cremini mushrooms, stemmed and halved**
- 2 **cloves garlic, minced**
- ½ **cup white wine**

• Preheat oven to 450°F.

• Lay out the sheets of parchment paper (or aluminum foil) on a flat work surface. Place a piece of fish in the center of each sheet, drizzle with a bit of olive oil, and season with salt on both sides. Top with a lemon slice and equal portions of the tomatoes, fennel, mushrooms, and garlic. Season the vegetables with salt and black pepper.

• Just before sealing the packets, add 2 tablespoons of white wine to each packet. To seal the packets, fold the paper or foil over the fish and roll up the edges to create a tight pouch. Place on a baking sheet and cook in the oven for 12–15 minutes, depending on how thick the fish is.

> 200 calories, 5 g fat, 3 g fiber, 24 g protein

THE ZERO BELLY BURGERS

The story of burgers in America is sort of like the story of Arnold Schwarzenegger in the Terminator movies. They started out as the ultimate buffed-up villains—big, beefy weapons of mass destruction. But then we found out some burgers could actually protect us from harm. The right protein—lean, grass-fed beef, chicken, turkey, or fish—partnered up with nutrient-filled vegetables and a bun that's not just empty carbs—actually makes for the perfect ZERO BELLY meal.

But that doesn't mean that any drive-through beef slinger or cheesy chain restaurant is doing burgers right. At Ruby Tuesday's, for example, you won't find a single burger with less than 1,200 calories—almost as much as you'll eat in a whole day of feasting on ZERO BELLY foods! And of course, from gluten-filled buns to corn-fed beef packed with saturated fat, most restaurant burgers should be limited to cheat meals only—and even then, consider the cheat to be of Madoffian proportions.

So when a burger reaches out its meaty hand and says, "Come with me if you want to live," how do you know if you should trust it? Just remember the three ZERO BELLY Questions:

• **Where's my protein?** This one's easy, of course. All burgers are protein packed. But the other two are trickier.

• **Where's my fiber?** Typical hamburger buns don't offer much, nor do the slice of bland tomato and iceberg lettuce that come on top. Choose a high-fiber, gluten-free bun (look for one made from healthy grains like brown rice, millet, amaranth, or buckwheat—not potato or tapioca starch) and stack it high with ZERO BELLY foods like leafy greens and colorful vegetables. I've included some great options, below. Or consider skipping the bun altogether and using a Romaine lettuce wrap or even a couple of Portobello mushroom caps.

• **Where's my healthy fat?** When you choose grass-fed beef, you're getting a meat that's almost as high in anti-inflammatory omega-3 fatty acids as some fish. (You are what you eat, and so is your cow.) Conventionally raised beef, which feeds on corn, is higher in saturated fat and inflammation-causing omega-6s. That's why grass-fed meats and fish make great ZERO BELLY burger fare. To up the ante, a generous slice of avocado always helps.

---

4 FAVORITE GLUTEN-FREE BUNS

Canyon GF Hamburger Buns

200 calories
4 g fat
4 g protein
4 g fiber

Canyon's hamburger buns are terrific tasting and feature ZB-approved ingredients like brown rice flour, whole grain millet, and sesame seeds.

Get Happy Campers Wild Buns

217 calories
0 g fat
4 g protein
3 g fiber

With a brand name like "Get Happy" and an organic ingredient list that reads like this— *whole millet seed, whole teff seed, whole buckwheat seed, whole quinoa seed, whole amaranth seed*—need I say more? I'm WHOLLY impressed.

Food for Life Brown Rice English Muffins

110 calories
1 g fat
1 g protein
2 g fiber

I love the texture contrast of a crusty, toasted English muffin with a tender, juicy burger. And Food for Life's Gluten Free Brown Rice variety is the "cleanest" on the market.

Manna Organic Ciao Chia Bread

2 slices: 160 calories,
4 g fat
2 g protein
2 g fiber

When the burger's the star, sometimes a couple of slices of thin crunchy toast is all you need. Made with organic brown rice flour and sprouted chia seeds, Manna's Ciao Chia variety is a belly-friendly favorite.

THE ZERO BELLY BURGER MATRIX

Calling all culinary ninjas! The recipes included in this book are taste-tested and nutritionally sound, but there are any number of ways you can mix, match, and customize the ZERO BELLY burger of your dreams. So get into the kitchen and create a dish that would make Bobby Flay beam with pride.

THE STAR! (Burger)

Ground turkey
Ground chicken
Ground beef
Salmon
Tuna
Chicken breast

THE VEHICLE! (Bun)

Gluten-free burger bun
Gluten-free English muffin
Gluten-free toast
Portobello caps
Lettuce leaves
(Romaine, Bibb)

THE SUPPORTING PLAYERS! (Veggie Toppings)

Lettuce
Arugula
Alfalfa sprouts
Cucumber
Avocado (1/4 per)
Fresh herbs
Tomato
Red onion
Shredded carrot
Roasted red peppers
Jalapeños
Caramelized onions
Sauteed mushrooms
Asian Slaw (see page 145)

THE EXTRAS! (Condiments; see starter kit on page 91 for best brands)

Ketchup
Mustard
Guacamole
Salsa
GF pickles
Wasabi mayo (see page 143)

THE ZERO BELLY BURGER RECIPES

THE ULTIMATE BURGER

Makes 4 servings

- 1 **pound ground 94%** (or leaner) **beef**
- 1 **teaspoon salt**
- 1 **teaspoon freshly cracked black pepper**
- 8 **ounces sliced mushrooms**
- $\frac{1}{2}$ **teaspoon extra-virgin olive oil**
- 4 **gluten-free hamburger buns**
- 2 **cups arugula**
- $\frac{1}{2}$ **cup Caramelized Onions** (see recipe opposite)
  Ketchup and mustard (optional)

• Heat a grill or stovetop grill pan until hot. Combine the beef, salt, and pepper in a bowl and gently mix. Form into 4 patties. *Caution:* overworking the meat or packing your patties too tightly can make tough burgers.

• Cook the burgers for 2–3 minutes and flip. Cook on the other side for another 2–3 minutes, until nicely charred on the outside but still medium-rare to medium within. (The center of the patty should be firm but easily yielding—like a Nerf football.)

• Meanwhile, sauté the sliced mushrooms in the olive oil until the mushrooms soften and release their liquid.

Divide the arugula among the buns and top with the burgers, onions, and mushrooms and 1 teaspoon each ketchup and mustard (optional).

> 387 calories, 13 g fat, 31 g protein, 6 g fiber

QUIRKY TURKEY BURGER

Makes 4 servings

- 1 pound lean 94–99% ground turkey
  Salt and pepper
- ½ red bell pepper, seeded and finely chopped
- 1 scallion, white part only, chopped
- 4 gluten-free hamburger buns
  Lettuce
  Tomato, sliced
- ½ avocado, sliced
  Ketchup and mustard (optional)

- Combine turkey, salt, and pepper in a large bowl. Add bell pepper and scallion and mix well.

- Form into 4 patties. Chill until ready to use.

- Heat a grill pan over medium-high heat. Cook burgers, turning once, until no longer pink in center, about 5 minutes per side.

- Place patties on toasted buns with lettuce, tomato, and avocado and 1 teaspoon each ketchup and mustard (optional).

> 362 calories, 15 g fat, 33 g protein, 3 g fiber

SECRET WEAPON:
Caramelized Onions

Properly caramelized onions take time, but make up a big batch and have them on hand for smothering burgers, covering sandwiches, and topping juicy hunks of grilled steak or fish. Cook at least 3 large red onions (remember, they'll shrink down as the water cooks out) in a large pot with ½ tablespoon of extra-virgin olive oil over a very low flame. Add a generous pinch of salt, which will help draw the moisture out. Cover the pot, removing the lid every 3 or 4 minutes to stir the onions. Cook for at least 20 minutes, up to 45 minutes, depending on how sweet you like your onions.

WHO YOU CALLIN' CHICKEN BURGER

Makes 4 servings

- 2 tablespoons mayonnaise
- 2 tablespoons chopped sundried tomatoes
  Juice of ½ lemon
- 2 cloves garlic, finely minced
- 1 teaspoon chopped fresh rosemary
  Salt and black pepper
- 1 pound lean ground chicken
- 4 gluten-free English muffins
- 2 cups arugula, baby spinach, or mixed greens

• In a mixing bowl, combine the mayonnaise, sundried tomatoes, lemon juice, garlic, and rosemary. Season with a pinch of salt and black pepper. Set the aioli aside.

• Preheat a grill, grill pan, or cast-iron skillet. Combine the ground chicken with ½ teaspoon salt and ½ teaspoon black pepper and mix gently. Without overworking the meat, form into four patties until the chicken just comes together.

• When the grill or skillet is hot (if using a skillet, add a touch of oil), add the burgers. Cook on the first side for 5 to 6 minutes, until a nice crust develops. Flip and cook for another 3 to 4 minutes, until the burgers are firm but ever so slightly yielding to the touch and cooked through. Remove the burgers. While the grill or pan is hot, toast the buns.

• Layer the toasted muffin bottoms with the arugula, top each with a burger, then slather the aioli over the top of each. Crown with the muffin tops and serve.

> 400 calories, 15 g fat, 24 g protein, 4 g fiber

HOT TUNA BURGERS

Makes 4 servings

- 1 pound fresh tuna
- 4 scallions, minced
- 1 teaspoon minced fresh ginger
- 1 tablespoon low-sodium soy sauce
- 1 teaspoon toasted sesame oil
- 2 teaspoons olive oil mayonnaise
- ½ tablespooon prepared wasabi (from powder or in premade paste)
- 4 gluten-free hamburger buns, lightly toasted
- 1 cup sliced cucumber
- 2 cups arugula

• Chop the tuna into ½" cubes, then place in the freezer for 10 minutes to firm up (this will make grinding easier).

• Working in batches if necessary, pulse the tuna in a food processor to the consistency of ground beef. (Be sure not to overdo it; you only want to pulse it enough so that you can form patties.) Transfer to a mixing bowl and mix in the scallions, ginger, soy sauce, and sesame oil. Form into four equal patties. Place in the fridge for at least 10 minutes to firm up before grilling.

• Preheat a well-oiled grill or grill pan. When hot, add the patties and cook for 2–3 minutes a side, until browned on the outside but still medium-rare in the center. Flip and handle carefully, as these burgers are more delicate than beef burgers.

• Mix the mayo with the wasabi, then spread evenly on the muffin tops. Line the bottoms with cucumber and arugula, top with the burgers, then crown with the muffin tops.

> 412 calories, 8 g fat, 31 g protein, 5 g fiber

TERIYAKI SALMON BURGERS

Makes 4 servings

> 1 pound salmon, finely chopped
> 1 egg
> ½ cup almond meal
> 4 scallions, thinly sliced
> 1 tablespoon low-sodium soy sauce
> Asian-style chili sauce like sriracha to taste
> 2 tablespoons teriyaki sauce, plus more for serving
> 4 gluten-free English Muffins, toasted
> 1 cup Asian Slaw (see opposite)

• Preheat a grill or grill pan over medium heat. Combine the salmon, egg, almond meal, scallions, soy sauce, and chili sauce in a bowl and mix thoroughly. Use your hands to gently form 4 patties. The patties will be very moist, but if the mixture is too dry it will be hard to form patties.

• Brush the tops of the burgers with about half the teriyaki sauce and place on the grill, sauce side down. Grill for about 4 minutes, until the burger firms up and easily pulls away from the grill. Brush the tops with the remaining teriyaki sauce and flip. Continue grilling for 4 minutes longer, until the burgers are cooked all the way through.

• Divide the burgers among the muffins, brush with a bit of additional teriyaki sauce, and top with generous piles of the slaw.

> 511 calories, 21 g fat, 33 g protein, 5 g fiber

ASIAN SLAW

Makes 4–6 servings

Juice of 1 lime
1 tablespoon mayonnaise
1 tablespoon honey
1 teaspoon Asian-style chili sauce like sriracha
1 teaspoon sesame oil
8 cups shredded cabbage
(preferably a mix of purple and napa cabbage)
1 large carrot, peeled and grated
1 tablespoon sesame seeds
Salt and pepper

• In a large salad bowl, mix together the lime juice, mayonnaise, honey, chili sauce, and sesame oil. Add the cabbage, carrot, and sesame seeds and toss to combine. Season with salt and pepper.

> 77 calories, 3 g fat, 2 g protein, 3 g fiber

SNACKS

ZERO BELLY COOKIES

Ripe banana acts both as the glue that holds these together as well as a major source of natural sweetness, while ground almonds stand in as a fiber- and protein-rich substitute for refined flour. Peanut butter and dark chocolate complete the package, adding healthy fat, antioxidants, and a double helping of deliciousness. The end result—nutty, sweet, chocolaty—is like a fresh slice of banana bread, in crunchy, chewy cookie form.

Makes 12 cookies

- 1 1/3 **cups unsalted blanched almonds**
- 2 **very ripe bananas**
- 1/3 **cup brown sugar**
- 1/2 **cup peanut butter**
- 1/2 **teaspoon baking soda**
- **Pinch of salt**
- 1/2 **cup vegan dark chocolate chips**

• Preheat oven to 350°F.

• Place the almonds in a food processor and pulse until ground to a near flour-like consistency.

• In a mixing bowl, mash the bananas into a paste. Add the brown sugar, peanut butter, baking soda, salt, and ground almonds and stir until evenly combined. Gently fold in the chocolate chips.

• Form each cookie by dropping 2 tablespoons of the batter onto a cookie sheet, leaving at least 3 inches between cookies. Bake for 8–10 minutes, until the edges are just brown.

> Per cookie: 114 calories, 8 g fat, 3.5 g protein, 2.5 g fiber

ALMOND, BROTHERS

Makes 4 snack-size servings

- 1 teaspoon extra virgin olive oil
- 1 clove garlic
- 1 tablespoon rosemary leaves
- 1 cup whole unsalted raw almonds or mixed nuts
  Salt to taste

• Heat the olive oil in a sauté pan over medium heat.
Add the garlic and rosemary and cook until the garlic is lightly browned. Add the almonds and cook, stirring occasionally, until lightly toasted and fragrant, about 5 minutes.
Season with salt to taste. Cool and store in a sealed container.

> 145 calories, 12.5 g fat, 5 g protein, 2.5 g fiber

APPLE AND NUT BUTTER

I love the classic apple and peanut butter pairing, but feel free to substitute any ZB fruit or vegetable.

- 1 small Pink Lady apple
- 1 tablespoon peanut or almond butter

> 150 calories, 8 g fat, 3 g protein, 5 g fiber

CHOCO-POPCORN

- 1 tablespoon popcorn kernels (2 cups popped)
- 1 teaspoon coconut oil for popping
  (melt first, toss kernels to coat)
- 1 square dark chocolate, melted
  (Ghirardelli Midnight Reverie is a good brand)

• Follow package directions for popcorn. Drizzle with melted chocolate and swoon.

> 143 calories, 11 g fat, 3 g fiber, 2 g protein

GROWN-UP GOLDFISH

8 gluten-free crackers (Blue Diamond Nut-Thins Cracker Snacks, Pecan is a good brand)
2 ounce smoked salmon (Echo Falls is a good brand)

> 155 calories, 6 g fat, 14 g protein, 2 g fiber

ZERO BELLY GRAB-AND-GO SNACKS

Some "nutrition bars" are actually worse for you than a Snickers—loaded with sugar, fat, low-quality soy protein, and enough artificial ingredients to make a chemist's head explode. Whole foods are always the preferred option. But, hey, life happens, and in a pinch, a nutrition bar can serve as a ZERO BELLY meal or snack replacement—if you choose wisely! Next time you're staring down an aisle of candy—er, nutrition bars—here are your safest bets:

KIND (all flavors)
LÄRABAR (all flavors)
Raw Revolution Organic Bars (all flavors)
Clif, Kit's Organic (all flavors)

CHAPTER NINE

THE ZERO BELLY WORK- OUTS

Full-Body Fitness Plans that Reveal Your Abs—Without Sit-ups!

Washboard abs. Six-pack abs. Sculpted abs. Shredded abs. Ripped abs. When it comes to exercising your stomach, sometimes it's hard to know whether you're talking about a body part or a heavy-duty kitchen appliance. I don't know about you, but the last thing I want to happen to my belly is for someone to rip it or shred it. Ouch!

As the editorial director of *Men's Fitness* and someone who's been researching, reporting on, and doing the best workouts in the world for more than twenty years, I've seen just about every abs exercise ever invented. So let me share with you a dirty little secret: The best way to get abs is to not waste a lot of time working your abs.

Whaaaat?

It's true. You don't need to be able to crack walnuts with your belly button in order to have a lean, flat, muscular stomach. What you need is a diet that melts visceral fat, and a workout that builds full-body fitness by focusing on lean muscle growth.

Well, I've already given you the diet. Now I want to share with you the workout. Seven of them, actually.

Do you have to try all seven? No.

Do you have to try any of them? No.

Do you ever have to lift anything heavier than this book or the tablet you might be reading it on? No.

Most "calorie in/calorie out" diets require you to either (a) eat almost nothing or (b) eat plenty but exercise like a madman. But that's not what ZERO BELLY is about.

My diet plan is designed to fight belly fat by reducing inflammation, improving digestion, and shutting down the fat storage system. It's not about burning off more calories than you take in. So it's unique in that exercise is merely an option.

That said, if you've come this far in the book, you surely have started to hate belly fat as passionately as I do. And you should be motivated to do everything in your power to bring it to its knees.

So why not try a workout?

FED UP WITH SIT-UPS!

Now, I don't want you to waste a lot of time on abs exercises. But if you think I'm recommending you don't work your core, you're wrong. Strong abdominal muscles are critical for everything from helping you retain correct posture to protecting you from back injury to making you look sweet in a sweater. In fact, if you were going to work only one body part, I'd recommend it be your abs—or core, or midsection, or whatever term you'd like. (In fact, in the next chapter, I've built for you a series of abs workouts that you can do in just seven minutes—perfect for days when you can't fit in a full-body training session.)

A few years back, Hugh Jackman—the actor who became a fitness icon by playing Wolverine in the X-Men movies—told a story about how he wrecked his back

playing sports as a teenager. He had grown really tall really fast, and one day he leapt up to catch a ball and tore a series of muscles along his spine. And what he learned from that experience was to always focus on having a strong core foundation—stronger abs lead to a stronger body, period.

But people like Hugh Jackman, whose careers depend on having lean, flat, defined stomachs, don't spend twenty minutes a day working their abs. They understand that if you want a flat, firm stomach and abs that show, you have to burn fat, and you have to build full-body muscle. And abs workouts are terrible at both.

There are two ways that exercise burns fat. The first is the obvious one: as you sweat your way through a workout, your body uses an elevated number of calories to power you along. Those calories are derived first from the glycogen stored in your muscles and then, as that becomes depleted, from the fat stored in your belly and elsewhere. And an abs workout simply isn't an efficient way to burn calories. Three sets of thirty sit-ups may be awkward, painful, and annoying, but calorie-burning? Not so much.

But the second and more significant way in which exercise helps lead to a ZERO BELLY is by increasing the amount of muscle in your body. In previous chapters, I outlined the war between muscle and fat that's going on, 24/7, inside your body. And you already know which side you want to win, right?

The more muscle you build, the more fat you'll burn—all day, every day, even when you're asleep—and the better chance you'll have of giving your abs a front-row seat. To do that, you need to work the most muscle tissue you can at the highest intensity possible. Think of exercise as an investment: if you were trying to figure out where to park your money, you'd want to pour the most into the investment that gives the highest yield. Same thing for your workout—put the most effort into the muscles that have the most tissue, and therefore the best opportunity for growth. And let's face it, your abdominal muscles are never going to be as big as, say, your butt muscles.

Now, what I've said so far might sound like a bit of a contradiction: we want to have strong abs, because strong abs are the foundation of fitness, but we don't want to waste a lot of time working the abs, because that's not going to help us get a lean, flat belly. Hmmm . . . a dilemma. Fortunately, I've got the solution right here.

THE FULL-BODY ABS WORKOUTS

That's right—the best way to burn fat, build muscle, *and* strengthen your core is a complete abs workout *without any actual abs exercises*!

That may sound impossible, but it's not. In fact, we use our abs for almost everything we do, and most of the time when you're exercising—whether you're running, lifting weights, practicing yoga, or dancing with the stars—you're working your abs. But there's one exception: our abs get a rest whenever we sit down. And guess what? A lot of workouts—especially weight workouts—involve sitting down. So here's your new abs mantra: don't sit up, stand up!

The following workouts are based on exercises that aren't supported by a seat, bench, or machine. Because the abdominals are part of a complex network of muscles that stabilize the midtorso against any and all forces that might compromise the spine (which, as we know, is bad), any time we do an exercise that requires the body to self-stabilize, the abs are brought into play. And since each of these workouts focuses on the big muscle groups of the body, you'll be burning the maximum number of calories and building the maximum amount of muscle.

These workouts are built on the concept of metabolic circuits, a combination of cardio and resistance training that strengthens the whole body while also burning as many calories as possible. Each is balanced to ensure that you work complementary muscle groups, giving one set of muscles a thorough workout, then letting them rest as you work a very different muscle group.

All of the workouts are built on the same structure: Each consists of a circuit of five "supersets," back-to-back exercises that target the same set of muscles in different ways. There's no rest between the two exercises in each superset, but a one-minute rest between each superset and a two-minute rest at the end of the circuit.

Are you saying, "Ah, that sounds easy. So much rest in the middle of the workout! Cool"? Well, I promise you, "easy" is not what you're going to feel about halfway through. In fact, you're going to hate me. I guarantee it. The combination of massive calorie burn and demands for muscle strength will have your whole body saying, "Whoa!"

Your belly fat will never know what hit it.

Each of the metabolic circuits in this chapter is designed with the same concept in mind: minimal equipment changes, to make the workout easy to perform, and minimal time investment, so you can get on with the business of life. Before we start, a few points:

Take it easy. The ZERO BELLY workouts are more demanding than they seem. Here are a few guidelines, based on your current fitness level:

- If you're not familiar with weights, start slow, and use much lighter weights than you think you'll need.

- If you're used to lifting weights, start slow, and use much lighter weights than you think you'll need.

- If you are the reigning Mr. Olympia and your biceps are larger than your head, start slow, and use much lighter weights than you think you'll need.

I'm not kidding here. You should get through the entire first circuit and wonder, "What's the big deal?" You won't be thinking that a circuit or two later. Use a weight that you can lift ten times with only modest effort.

Take it easy, part two. While each workout is designed as a set of five circuits, don't try to do all five in your first session. It's more important to keep proper form and stick to the timing of the workout. Do only two or three circuits your first time out, and work up to the point where you can do five. Once you can do five circuits and still have a little energy to spare at the end, increase the weight for each exercise modestly.

Don't sit down. While there are plenty of breaks built into each circuit, you want your abs always on duty, always working to support you. So stay standing during the rest periods. (Besides, if you sit down, there's a chance you might not want to get back up again!) Remember, don't sit up, stand up!

Drink. This workout rapidly depletes your hydration, so make sure you have a water bottle at the ready throughout the workout. And remember to follow up your training session with a special ZERO BELLY postworkout drink for optimal results!

Do what you feel. The great thing about ZERO BELLY workouts is that you can do any one you want, depending on where you are, what you feel like, and which equipment is being hogged by the gym rats. Hit the floor, make a choice, and go for it!

Good luck. And remember: don't hate me.

THE ZERO BELLY FULL-BODY CHALLENGE

More than five hundred men and women signed up for the original ZERO BELLY Challenge, and you've met many of them earlier in this book.

Not only did they find amazing results through the diet plan alone, but many of them also incorporated this specially designed dumbbell workout into their fitness plan three times a week.

Select a set of light dumbbells that you can press overhead from a standing position ten times. You can use this weight for the entire circuit, or increase the weight for some exercises as you become more familiar with the program. You'll do each two-part superset of exercises without resting at all in between. Then after each superset, you'll rest for sixty seconds before tackling the next. Once you've completed all four supersets, rest for two minutes. Try to do two circuits on your first go-round, and work up to five circuits as you get stronger, fitter, and leaner!

This circuit is written to include dumbbells, but it can be performed without weight, with a barbell (or even water bottles or a broomstick), depending on your strength and fitness level.

Perform this circuit at least three times a week with at least one day of rest in between each circuit.

THE ZERO-BELLY FULL-BODY CHALLENGE

SUPERSET #1

1a. Dumbbell Shoulder Press (for a variation, use a barbell)

1b. Bent-Over Dumbbell Row

REST: 60 seconds

SUPERSET #2

2a. Dumbbell Squat (for a variation, use a barbell)

2b. Stiff-Legged Dumbbell Deadlift (for a variation, use a barbell)

REST: 60 seconds

SUPERSET #3

3a. Dumbbell Walking Lunge (10–12 each leg)

3b. Push-up (resting on your knees instead of your toes if you have to; plyo if advanced)

REST: 60 seconds

SUPERSET #4

4a. Step-up with Knee Raise (with or without dumbbells or barbell)

4b. Mountain Climbers

REST: 2 minutes.

Repeat the circuit 3 more times!

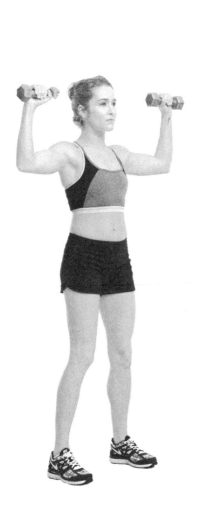
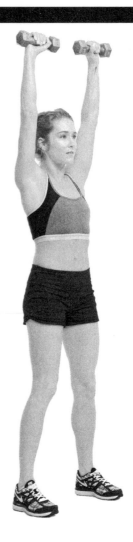

1a. DUMBBELL SHOULDER PRESS

Hold a dumbbell in each hand. Plant your feet firmly about hip width apart. Bend your elbows and position the dumbbells to each side of shoulders at ear level, making sure to rotate your wrists so that the palms of your hands are facing forward. This is your starting position.

Now, exhale as you push the dumbbells upward until they nearly touch at the top. Then, after a brief pause at the top contracted position, slowly lower the weights back down to the starting position while inhaling. Repeat for 10 repetitions.

1b. BENT-OVER DUMBBELL ROW

Plant your feet firmly about hip width apart. With a dumbbell in each hand (palms facing each other), bend your knees slightly and bring your torso forward by bending at the waist; as you bend make sure to keep your back straight until it is at a 60-degree angle. The weights should hang directly in front of you as your arms hang perpendicular to the floor. This is your starting position.

While keeping the torso stationary, bend your elbows and lift the dumbbells to your side (as you exhale), keeping your arms close to the body. On the top contracted position, squeeze the back muscles and hold for a second. Slowly lower the weights again to the starting position as you inhale. Repeat for 10 repetitions.

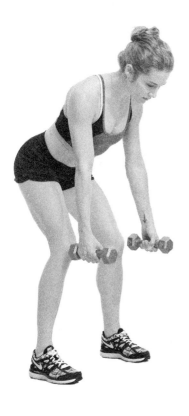
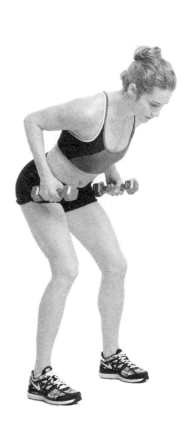

2a. DUMBBELL SQUAT

Stand up straight while holding a dumbbell in each hand (palms facing the sides of your legs). Position your legs using a shoulder-width medium stance with the toes slightly pointed out. Keep your head up at all times (looking down will throw you off balance), and also maintain a straight back. This will be your starting position.

Begin to slowly lower your torso by bending the knees and sitting back with the weight in your heels so that you maintain a straight posture with your head up. Continue down until your thighs are parallel to the floor. If you performed the exercise correctly, the front of the knees should make an imaginary perpendicular straight line with the toes. If your knees are past your toes, you're placing undue stress on the knee. Begin to raise your torso as you exhale by pushing the floor mainly with the heel of your foot as you straighten the legs again and go back to the starting position. Repeat for 10 repetitions.

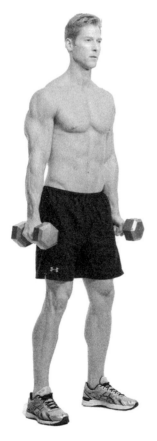
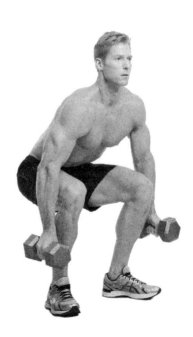

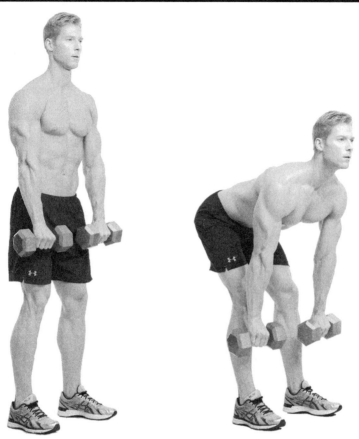

2b. STIFF-LEGGED DUMBBELL DEADLIFT

Hold a couple of dumbbells in front of your thighs, palms facing you. Stand with your torso straight and your legs spaced at a shoulder-width or narrower stance. The knees should be slightly bent. This is your starting position.

Keeping the knees stationary, lower the dumbbells down your legs toward your feet, keeping your legs straight but not locked, by bending at the waist while keeping your back straight. Keep moving forward, as if you were going to pick something up from the floor, until you feel a stretch on the hamstrings. Exhale as you perform this movement. Start bringing your torso up straight again by extending your hips and waist until you are back at the starting position.

Repeat for 10 repetitions.

3a. DUMBBELL WALKING LUNGE

Begin standing with your feet shoulder width apart and hold a couple of dumbbells by your side at arm's length. Step forward with one leg, flexing the knees to drop your hips. Descend until your rear knee nearly touches the ground. Your torso should remain upright, and your front knee should stay perpendicular to the front foot. Raise yourself back up to the starting position while keeping the weight on your heel. Step forward with your rear foot, repeating the lunge on the opposite leg. Repeat 10 lunges on each leg.

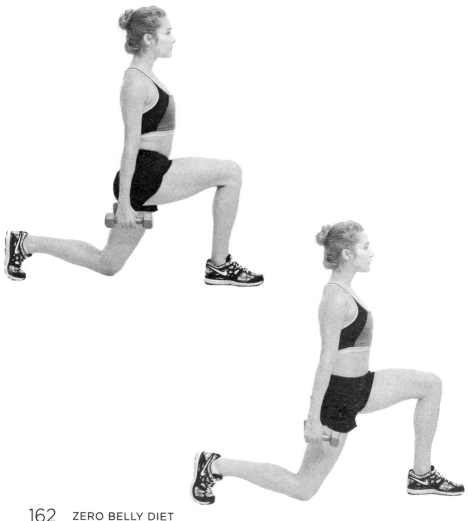

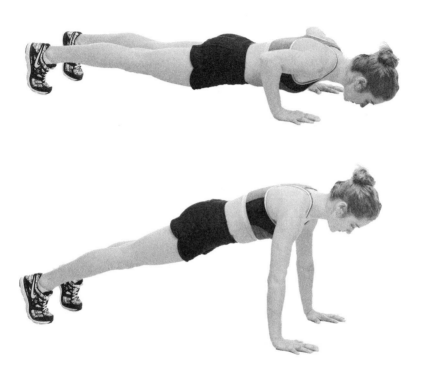

3b. PUSH-UP

Lie on the floor facedown with your hands at your sides, just outside your shoulders, and your feet hip-width apart. Raise your hips, thighs, and chest off the floor so your weight is supported by your toes and palms. This is the starting position. Exhale as you straighten your arms and push your body up until your arms are straight. Try to keep your head, hips, and ankles aligned as though your body is a straight plank. After a brief pause at the top, inhale as you lower yourself down. Repeat for 10 repetitions.

SUPERSET #4

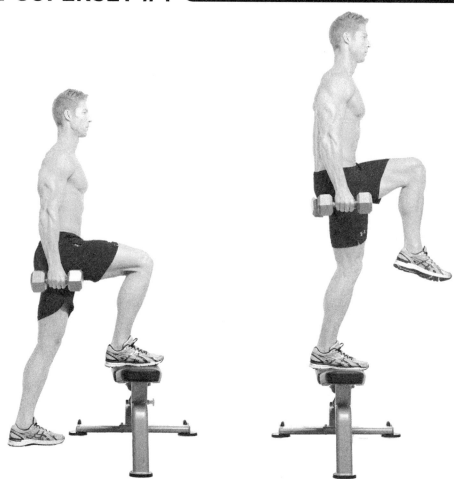

4a. STEP-UP WITH KNEE RAISE

Stand facing a box or bench about shin-high, with your feet at hip width and parallel to one another. Step up with your right foot and place it firmly on the top of the bench. This is your starting position. Now shift your weight to your right foot as you push off your right heel, straightening your right leg while simultaneously driving your left knee upward. At the top of the movement, you should be standing on your right leg atop the bench with your left thigh perpendicular to your body and parallel to the floor. Reverse the motion as you step back with your left leg to plant it on the floor behind you. Step your right foot off the bench and plant it on the floor so your feet are parallel again. Repeat the movement on the opposite side, stepping up onto the bench with your left leg and driving your right knee into the air. Repeat the sequence 10 times on each side.

Variation: Add dumbbells (as shown), or increase the box height to increase the difficulty of this exercise.

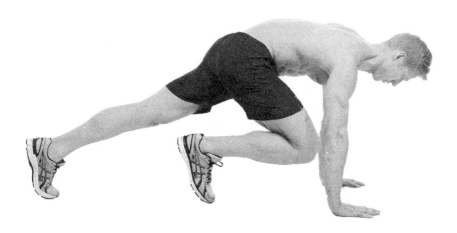

4b. MOUNTAIN CLIMBERS

Get onto all fours, with your weight supported by your hands and toes. Flex your left knee and hip as you bend the right leg, bringing your knee to your right elbow. Explosively reverse the positions of your legs, extending the right leg back into a straight position, supported by the toe, and bringing the left knee up to your left elbow simultaneously. Repeat in an alternating fashion for 10 repetitions on each side.

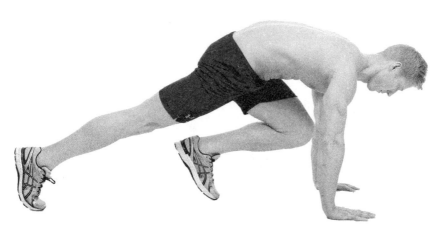

THE
ZERO
BELLY
BARBELL
WORKOUT

The barbell is the most basic piece of equipment in what gym rats call progressive resistance training but most folks call weight lifting. Nothing could be simpler than a bar with weights slipped over its ends, but it's the barbell's simple elegance that makes it such an invaluable device for exercising the body. The following workout utilizes only a barbell to work not only the entire body directly but the abdominals indirectly, too. It consists of a circuit of three supersets repeated four times. There's no rest between the two exercises in each superset, but a one-minute rest between each superset and a two-minute rest between circuits.

This workout should take you less than twenty minutes to complete, but if you're doing it right, you should feel thoroughly fatigued by the time you're finished!

THE ZERO BELLY BARBELL WORKOUT

Exercise	Reps	Rest
SUPERSET #1		
1a. Standing Press	10	None
1b. Barbell Push-up	10	30 sec
SUPERSET #2		
2a. Bent-Over Row (overhand grip)	10	None
2b. Barbell Plank	30 sec hold	30 sec
SUPERSET #3		
3a. Reverse Lunge	10 each leg	None
3b. Bent-Over Row (underhand grip)	10	120 sec

Repeat the circuit 3 more times for a total of 4!

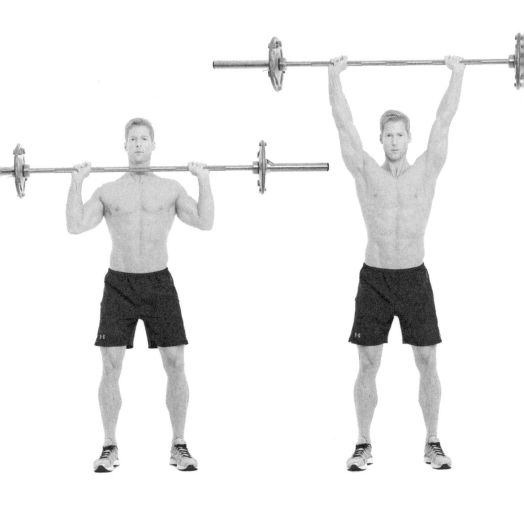

1a. STANDING PRESS

Place a barbell on a rack set to shoulder level. Grasp the bar with an overhand grip, hands slightly wider than your shoulders. Lift the bar off the rack and hold it in front of you at shoulder height. This is the starting position. Now press the bar straight overhead, remembering to keep your back tight and your eyes focused straight ahead or slightly higher. At the top of the lift, your arms should be completely straight. Bring the bar back to the starting position and repeat for a total of 10 reps.

1b. BARBELL PUSH-UP

This is the same as a standard push-up, except instead of putting your hands on the floor, you'll instead grasp the shaft of a barbell set on the floor. Be careful, as the bar will want to roll out. Your job is to keep your stomach muscles tight in order to keep the barbell in place as you perform your push-ups.

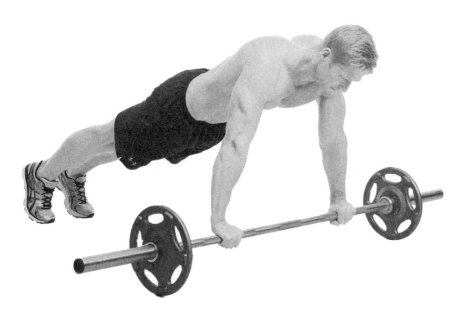

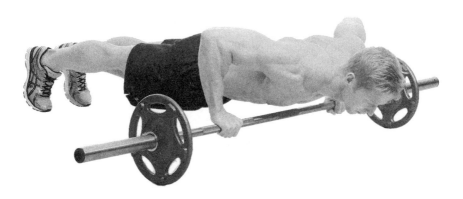

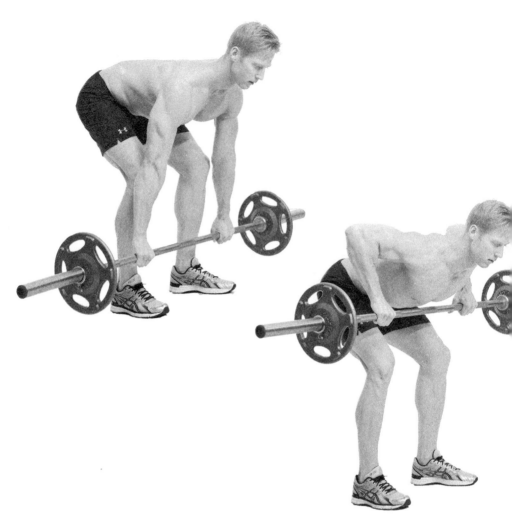

2a. BENT-OVER ROW (overhand grip)

Place a barbell on the floor in front of you and bend at the hips with knees slightly flexed so you can reach down to grasp the bar. Grip the bar with an overhand grip, with your hands slightly wider than your shoulders. Straighten your back and angle your hips so your torso is angled a few degrees above parallel with the floor. This is the starting position. Now drive your elbows back as you pull the barbell up to a point just below your sternum. Squeeze your shoulder blades together at the top of the movement, then lower the bar back down to complete a rep. Get a good stretch at the bottom of each rep and a good squeeze at the top.

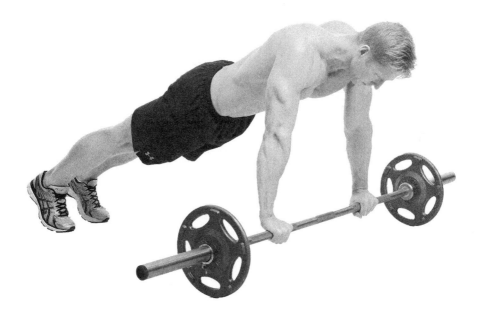

2b. BARBELL PLANK

Place a barbell on the floor and assume a push-up position, with your hands about shoulder width apart. Your body should be as stiff and straight as a plank, forming a straight line from head to toe. Again, there's an added degree of difficulty as you work to prevent the barbell from rolling out from under you. Hold the position for 30 seconds.

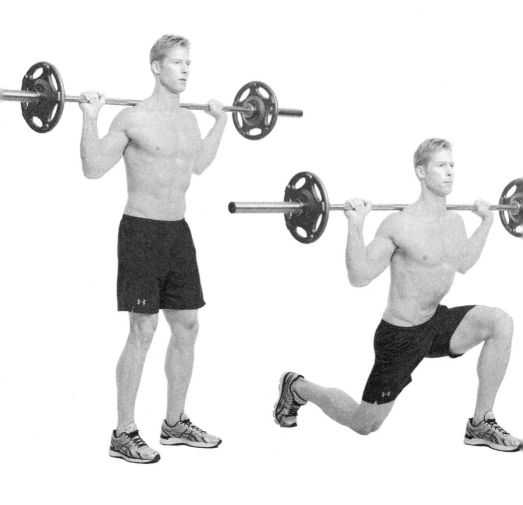

3a. REVERSE LUNGE

Place a barbell across your shoulders, as though you were carrying pails of water. Take a large step backward with one foot,
keeping your back flat and your eyes fixed straight ahead. Now
lower yourself in a split position until the knee of your rear leg
brushes the floor. Raise yourself back up to a standing position,
then step back with the opposite leg and repeat the sequence.
Continue alternating like this until you've performed 10 reps for
each leg.

3b. BENT-OVER ROW (underhand grip)

Follow the directions for the Bent-Over Row (overhand grip) on page 170, except reverse your grip so that your palms are underneath the bar.

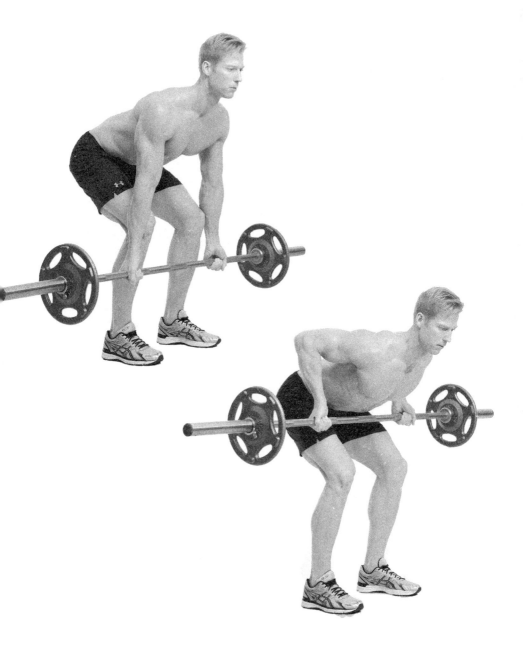

THE ZERO BELLY DUMBBELL WORKOUT

Dumbbells hold one distinct advantage over their cousin the barbell. Because your hands aren't fixed in relation to each other, as with a barbell, dumbbells give the advantage of being able to work each side of your body independently of the other. That means your hardworking right arm can't sneak in and help your slacker left arm out—so you get strong all over.

You'll need a bench and a pair of dumbbells for this workout. It should take you around twenty minutes to complete. Remember to start with a weight you can handle for 10 clean reps. That means no jerking motions—focus on form!

THE ZERO BELLY DUMBBELL WORKOUT

Exercise	Reps	Rest
SUPERSET #1		
1a. Sprinter	10 each side	None
1b. Reverse Lunge	10 each side	60 sec
SUPERSET #2		
2a. Standing Dumbbell Press	10	None
2b. Dumbbell Plank	30 sec hold	30 sec
SUPERSET #3		
3a. Standing Triceps Press	10	None
3b. Dumbbell Swing	10	120 sec

Repeat the circuit 3 times!

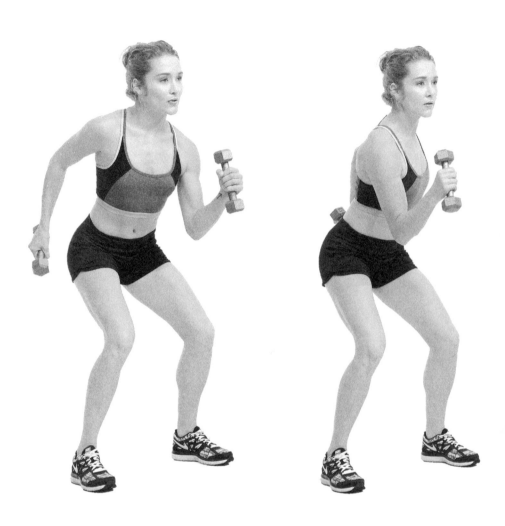

1a. SPRINTER

Stand with your feet together and hold a light dumbbell in each hand. Crouch down until your knees are bent to about 45 degrees. Now swing your arms back and forth in an alternating fashion. You're basically mimicking a sprinting motion without moving your legs. Although the movement will appear as if you are swinging the weights, make sure to control the motion, using only a little momentum to ensure steady motion. Alternate until you have completed 10 reps with each arm, for a total of 20.

1b. REVERSE LUNGE

Stand with your arms at your sides, holding a dumbbell in each hand. Take a large step backward with one foot, keeping your back flat and your eyes fixed straight ahead. Now lower yourself in a split position until the knee of your rear leg brushes the floor. Raise yourself back up to a standing position, then step back with the opposite leg and repeat the sequence. Continue alternating like this until you've performed the prescribed number of reps for each leg.

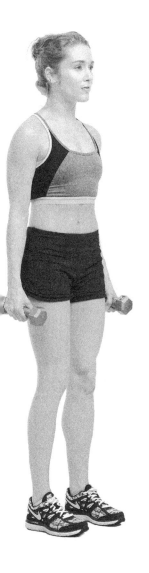
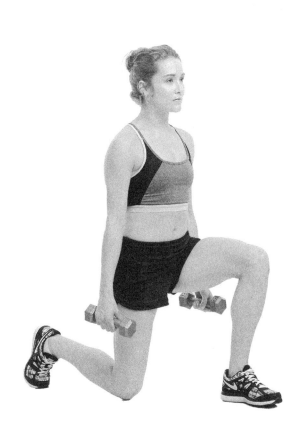

SUPERSET #2

2a. STANDING DUMBBELL PRESS

Grasp two dumbbells and hold them in front of you at shoulder height, palms facing each other. Press the dumbbells straight up as you rotate your arms; at the top of the motion, your palms should be facing out and your elbows straight. Keep your eyes focused straight ahead or slightly higher. Now lower the weights back down to the front of your shoulders, rotating them back to the starting position.

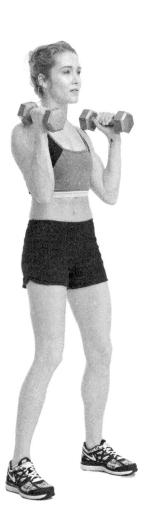
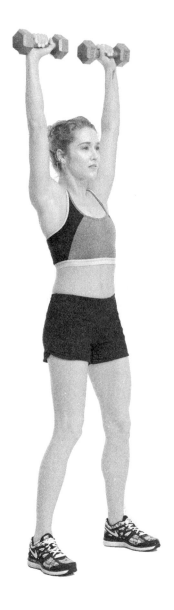

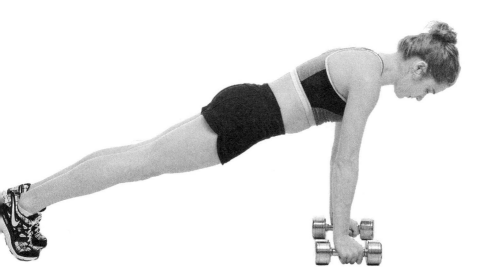

2b. DUMBBELL PLANK

Place two dumbbells on the floor and assume a push-up position, with your hands on the dumbbells about shoulder width apart. Your body should be as stiff and straight as a plank, forming a straight line from head to toe. There's an added degree of difficulty as you work to prevent the dumbbells from rolling out from under you. Hold the position for 30 seconds.

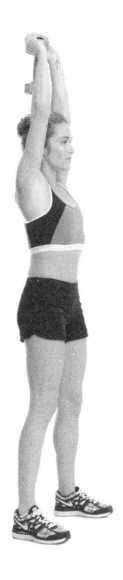
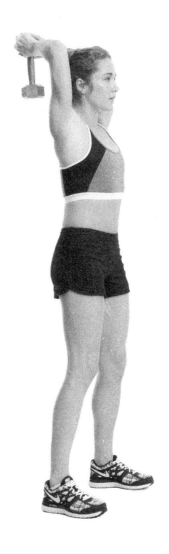

3a. STANDING TRICEPS PRESS

Stand with your feet shoulder-width apart. Grasp the head of a
dumbbell with both hands and extend your arms until they are
straight above your head. This is the starting position. Keeping
your upper arms still, inhale as you bend your elbows to lower
the weight behind your head. You should feel a stretch in your
triceps. Exhale as you press the weight back up to the starting
position in a smooth, arcing motion.

3b. DUMBBELL SWING

Grasp the handle of a dumbbell between both hands. Stand with your feet shoulder-width apart. With arms and back straight, squat down. Rise back into a standing position as you swing the dumbbell up and forward in front of you. At its highest point, the dumbbell should be aligned with the top of your head. Let the dumbbell swing back between your legs before using its momentum to propel it forward again.

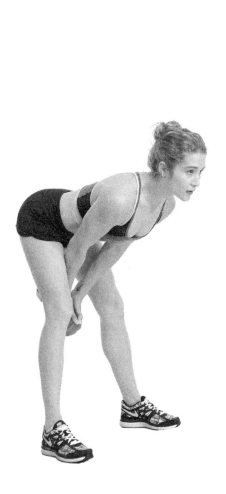
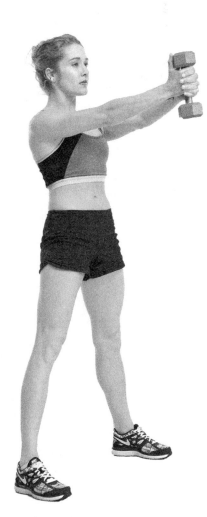

THE ZERO BELLY SUSPENSION WORKOUT

The suspension trainer is a simple yet superfunctional piece of equipment that was originally designed by former Navy SEAL Randy Hetrick. Randy found it tough to get in workouts while on the road: he couldn't very well carry a barbell or a pair of dumbbells with him on special assignments. Putting his sewing skills to the test, he fashioned what would become the prototype for the modern-day TRX out of an old jiujitsu belt and parachute webbing. That was in 1988. Today, the TRX suspension training system is a worldwide phenomenon and has spawned a number of similar products.

For this particular workout, any quality suspension trainer will do. The workout is designed to target your entire body with every exercise, with your core being a big part of it.

THE ZERO BELLY SUSPENSION TRAINER WORKOUT

Exercise	Time	Rest
1. Sprinter Start	30 sec each leg	60 sec
2. Squat	30 sec	60 sec
3. Hamstring Curl	30 sec	60 sec
4. Incline Push-up	30 sec	60 sec
5. Row	30 sec	60 sec
6. Rear Lateral	30 sec	60 sec
7. Kneeling Rollout	30 sec	60 sec
8. Curl	30 sec	60 sec
9. Straight Arm Plank	30 sec	60 sec
10. Crunch	30 sec	60 sec

Perform entire circuit once.

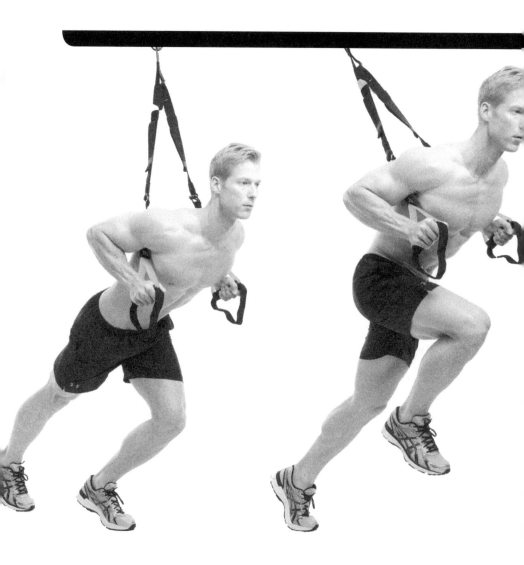

1. SPRINTER START

Grab the handles and hold them to your sides at chest height. The straps should be set to a length that allows you to lean forward enough to resemble the angle your body would be at when starting a sprint. Take a staggered foot stance and bring your rear knee forward and up, as if you were running, and then back. Repeat for 30 seconds, then switch feet and perform the movement with the opposite leg.

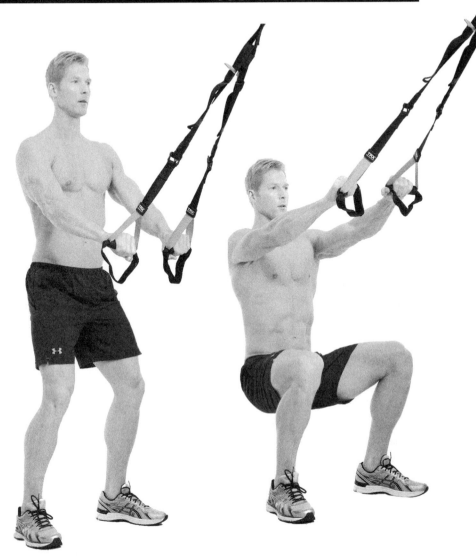

2. SQUAT

Holding the suspension handles firmly at about hip height, and with the straps pulled taut for stability, plant your feet firmly on the floor, set at about shoulder width apart. With back flat, squat down until your upper legs just pass the line where they're parallel with the floor, then rise back up to the full standing position. Repeat for 30 seconds.

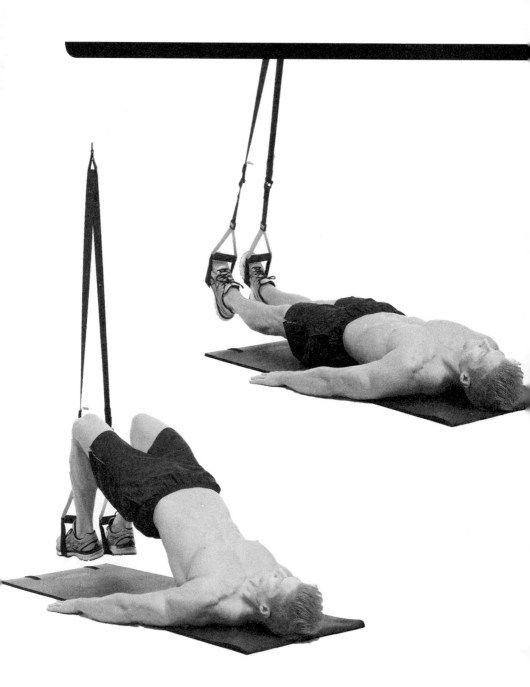

3. HAMSTRING CURL

Lie on your back with your legs straight and your soles firmly pressed into suspension handles. With your arms at your sides and your palms pressed against the floor, bring your knees in while raising your pelvis up until your lower legs are perpendicular to the floor. Slowly return to the starting position and repeat.

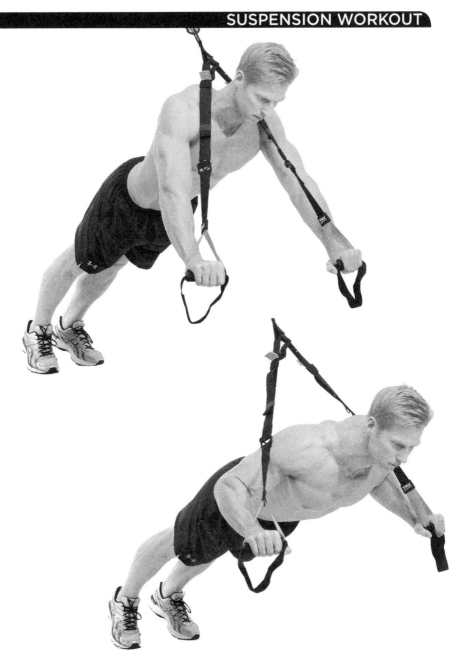

4. INCLINE PUSH-UP

Set the suspension trainer handles to anywhere from a foot to several feet off the ground, depending on your strength. Grab the handles and perform a push-up, making sure to keep the handles stable. The higher you set the handles, the easier the exercise becomes.

5. ROW

Stand facing the suspension straps, grab the handles, and with feet firmly planted, lean back until your arms are fully extended. With back flat, drive your elbows back to pull yourself forward. Slowly extend your arms again and repeat. The length to which you set the straps and the distance you stand from the unit where the straps are hung will determine the difficulty of the exercise.

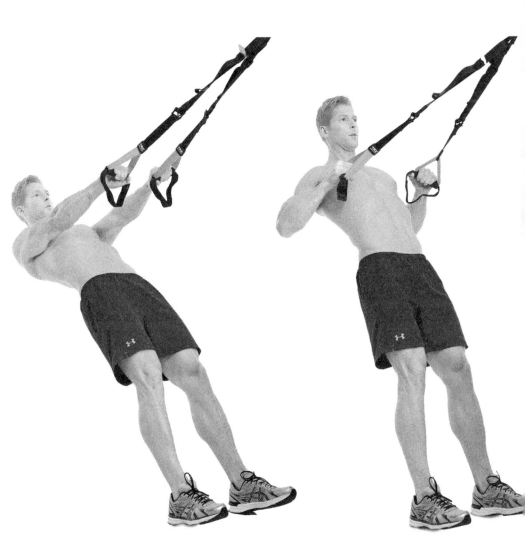

6. REAR LATERAL

Stand in a position similar to that of the row, except slightly farther from the straps, as this is a more challenging exercise. Lean back until your arms are fully extended and directly in front of you. Now, arc your arms out to your sides in a reverse hugging motion, bringing your body forward, until your hands are in line with your torso. Slowly return to the starting position and repeat.

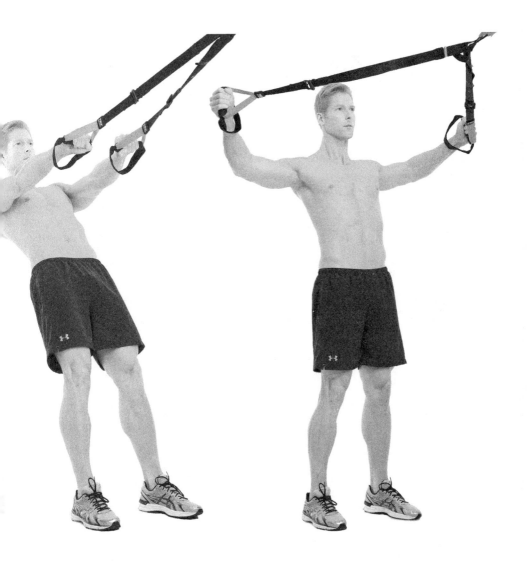

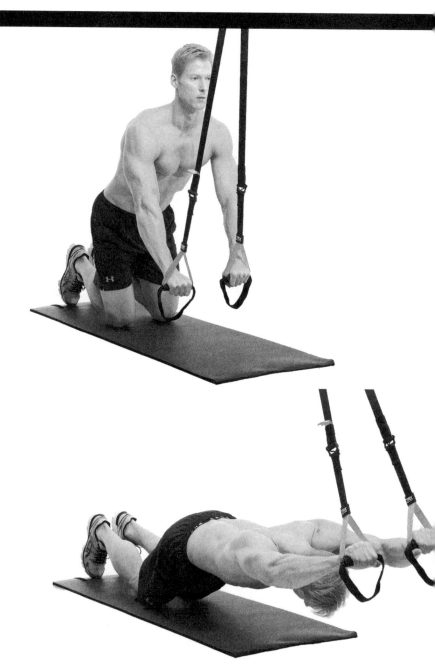

7. KNEELING ROLLOUT

Kneel on a pad in front of the suspension straps with the handles set very low to the ground. Grab the handles and push them forward until your arms and torso form a straight line, then retract your body again to complete a full rep.

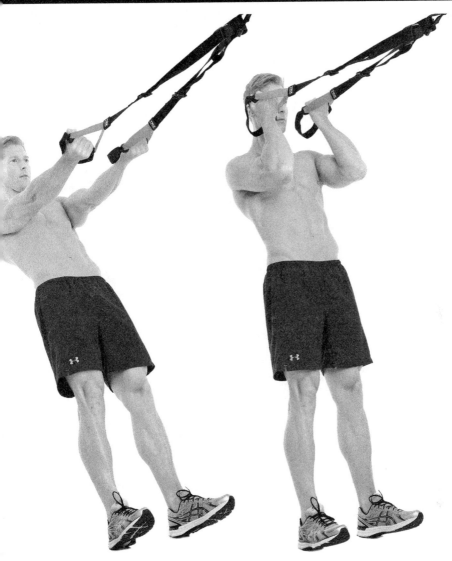

8. CURL

Stand facing the straps, a few feet away from them. Grab the handles with an underhand grip and lean back until your body is straight at anywhere from a 45-degree to 60-degree angle to the floor. Pull your body toward the handles, bending at the elbows, until your arms are bent at 90 degrees. Return to the starting position to complete one rep.

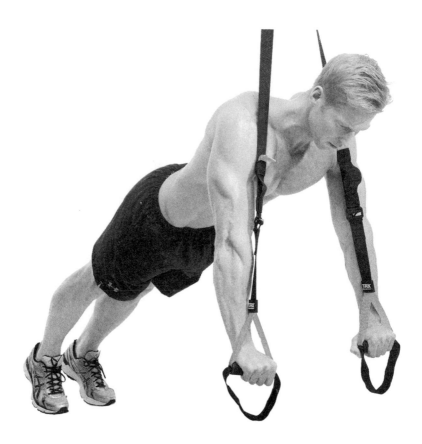

9. STRAIGHT-ARM PLANK

Set the handles to their lowest position and assume a push-up
position, with your arms extended and your body as straight as
a plank from head to toe. Controlling the motion of the straps is
key here. If it proves too difficult at first, try the exercise from a
kneeling position.

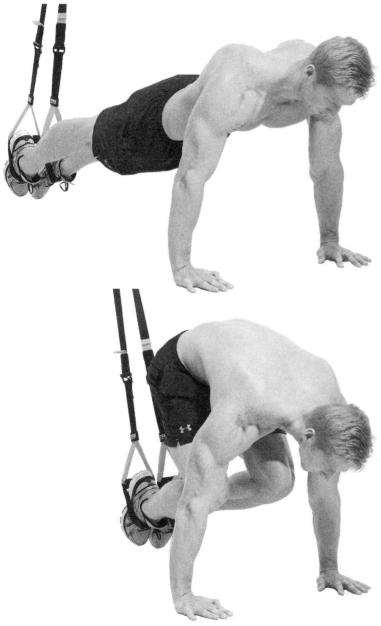

10. CRUNCH

Kneel facing away from the suspension straps, then hook the tops of your feet into the handles, which should be set to their lowest position (about a foot off the floor). Pull your knees toward your chest and then push them back out until your legs are straight to complete one rep.

THE ZERO BELLY HIIT BODY-WEIGHT WORKOUT

There's one piece of equipment absolutely everyone owns, regardless of income or level of commitment to the fitness life-style: your body. And it's a pretty wondrous piece of equipment at that. Believe it or not, it's possible to get in an intense work-out that will not only work all of your major muscle groups (core included) but burn fat and increase your cardio capacity as well—all while using no equipment at all.

This workout is based upon the HIIT training protocol, which has been the subject of a lot of research over the last couple of decades. HIIT stands for High Intensity Interval Training, and it involves short bursts of intense activity divided by rest periods half as long as the activity period. While traditional HIIT workouts are often performed on stationary bikes, this one involves body-weight exercises, thus maximizing aerobic efficiency while working the muscles of the entire body as well. This workout is surprisingly intense—so intense that four sessions of just four minutes of it per week will do the trick!

THE ZERO BELLY HIIT BODY-WEIGHT WORKOUT

Every exercise is to be performed as fast as possible without losing form.

3 minutes: Warm up on a stationary cardio machine, do jumping jacks, or jog in place

20 seconds: Run in Place (high knees)

10 seconds: Rest

20 seconds: Mountain Climbers

10 seconds: Rest

20 seconds: Skater Jumps (side-to-side, mimicking a skater's stride)

10 seconds: Rest

20 seconds: Push-ups (elbows close to sides of body)

10 seconds: Rest

Repeat work/rest cycle once

3 minutes: Cool down with any of the above warm-up movements

1. WARM-UP: JUMPING JACKS

Stand with your feet slightly less than shoulder width apart, hands at your sides. Jump into the air, spreading your feet as wide as you can while swinging your arms out to the sides and bringing your hands up over your head, palms facing forward. Immediately jump back up and return your hands and feet to the starting position. That's one Jumping Jack. Repeat at a comfortable pace without stopping for the duration of your warm-up.

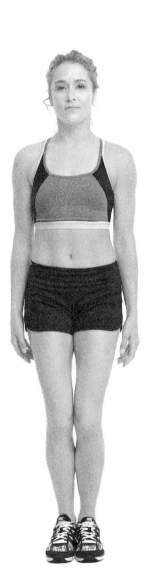
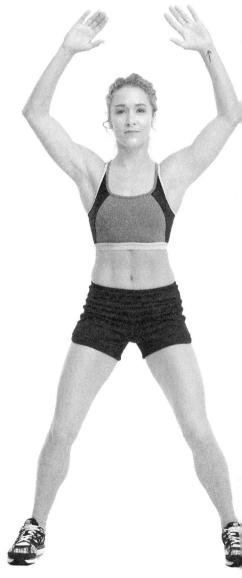

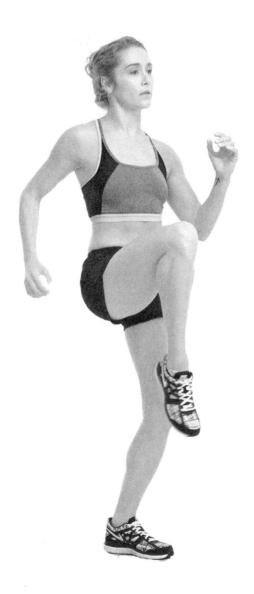

2. RUN IN PLACE (high knees)

Run in place, bringing your knees up as high as you can and pumping your legs as quickly as you can, for 20 seconds.

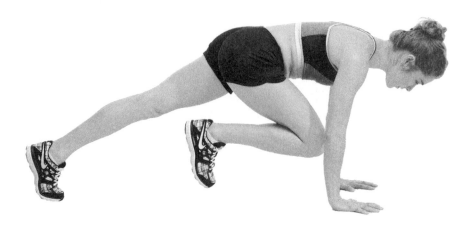

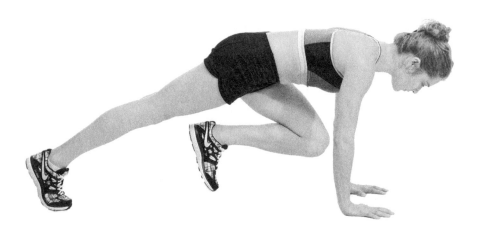

3. MOUNTAIN CLIMBERS

Get into a push-up position, with your arms straight. Raise your hips as you bring one knee up toward your chest, then quickly reverse leg position as you bring the other knee forward. The movement should be dynamic: rather than simply moving one leg followed by the other, get a rhythm going akin to jogging, where both feet are off the floor for a brief moment.

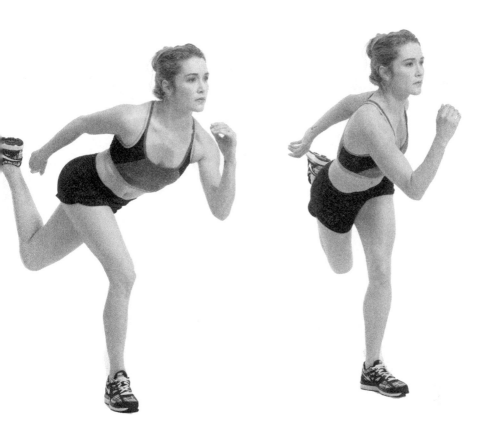

4. SKATER JUMPS

From a crouched position with your feet close together, take a sideways leap to your left, landing on your left foot, with your right foot sweeping behind it, your right arm sweeping in front of your midsection, and your left arm sweeping out to the side. Now hop to your right, landing on your right foot and reversing the position of your other limbs. This should be a smooth, comfortable motion that mimics the movement of a speed skater in action.

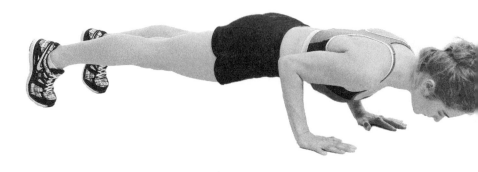

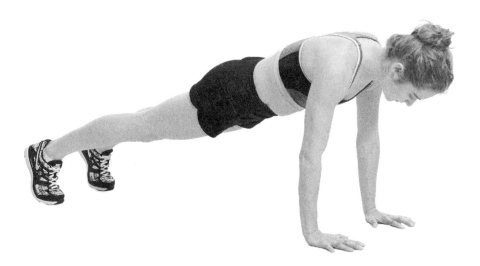

5. PUSH-UPS

Lie on the floor facedown with your hands at your sides, just outside your shoulders, and your feet hip-width apart. Raise your hips, thighs, and chest off the floor so your weight is supported by your toes and palms. This is the starting position. Exhale as you straighten your arms and push your body up until your arms are straight. Try to keep your head, hips, and ankles aligned as though your body is a straight plank. After a brief pause at the top, inhale as you lower yourself down. Repeat for 10 repetitions.

THE ZERO BELLY KETTLEBELL WORKOUT

Kettlebells are those cannonball-like weights with the handles on top that look so incredibly dangerous when someone else is swinging them around. In your hands, though, they're loaded weapons against flab.

Do this workout as a circuit, going through each exercise in order with no rest between, then rest for three minutes before starting over again. Five circuits is all it takes to get the job done.

THE ZERO BELLY KETTLEBELL WORKOUT

Exercise	Reps
1. Swing	10
2. Renegade Row	5 each side
3. Goblet Squat	10
4. One-Arm Clean and Press	5 each side

1. SWING

Take a wider-than-shoulders stance with back flat and ham-strings and glutes engaged, then bend at the knees to pick up a kettlebell placed between your feet. Using your arms as hooks, thrust your hips out and swing the kettlebell out in front of you until it reaches shoulder height. Let it swing back down as you guide it between your legs. Use the momentum created by the return swing to power the bell upward again once it comes back between your legs. This is a tricky movement that is dependent on flow, so don't force it.

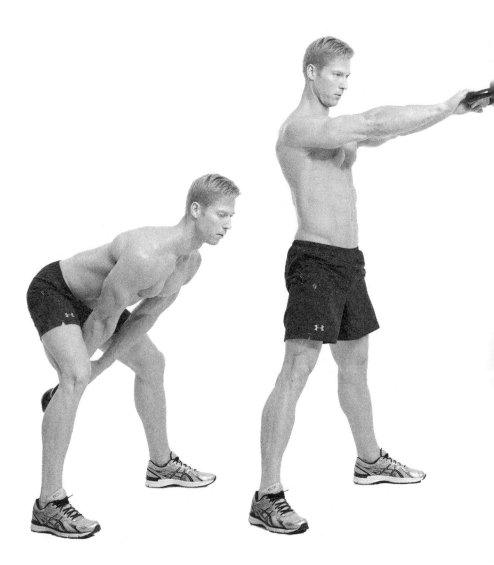

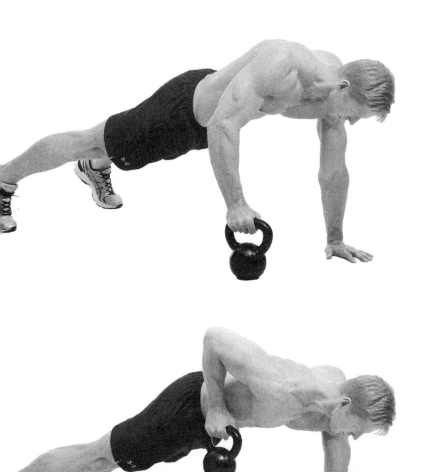

2. RENEGADE ROW

Get into a straight-arm plank position with your left palm on the floor and your right hand grasping the handle of a kettle-bell. Turn the handle so it's aligned with your torso. Shifting your weight onto your left arm, inhale as you pull the kettlebell straight up toward your rib cage. Exhale as you lower it back to the floor. Perform 5 reps, then switch hands and perform another 5 reps with your left hand.

3. GOBLET SQUAT

Hold a kettlebell with both hands on the sides of its handle up against your chest. With your feet set wider than your shoulders and your toes pointing slightly out, squat down until your upper legs are below parallel with the floor, keeping your back straight and eyes straight ahead throughout the movement. Rise up in a smooth motion to complete the rep.

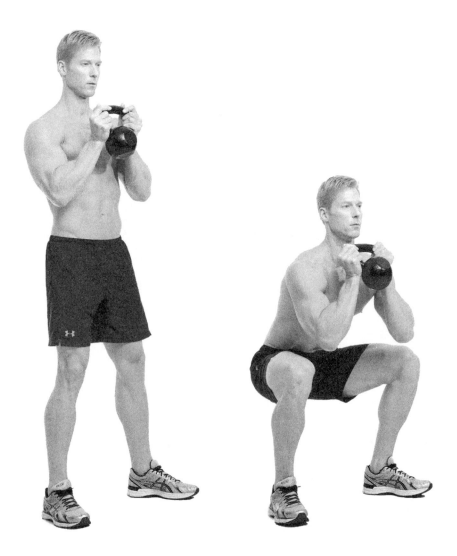

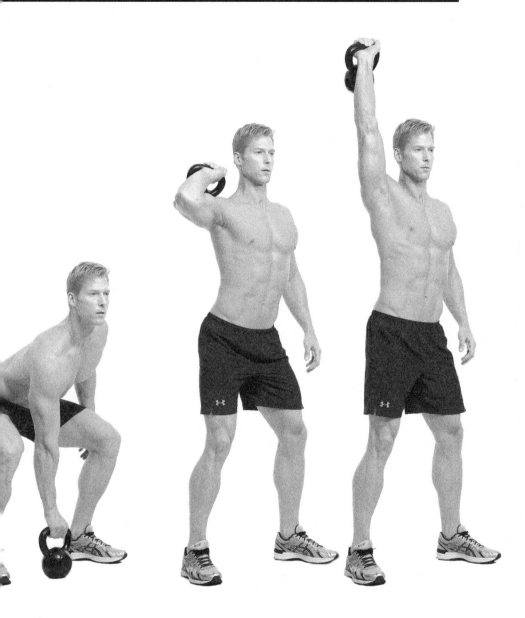

4. ONE-ARM CLEAN AND PRESS

Take a wider-than-shoulders stance with a kettlebell placed between your feet. Bending at the knees, and with your back straight, hoist the bell to shoulder height, letting the ball flip over so that it rests against the back of your shoulder. From there, press the kettlebell straight up, with the ball resting against your forearm. Return the bell to your shoulder, then back again to the floor to complete one rep.

THE ZERO BELLY SWISS BALL WORKOUT

Swiss balls are deceptive. Big, rubbery air-filled balls, they look soft and comfy, and they are—if all you do is sit on them. Employ them as part of your fitness routine, however, and you have a highly effective weapon in your battle against the bulge. The trick is to use their inherent instability to your advantage. As you work to stabilize yourself against the ball's natural tendency to roll, you activate a host of muscles, both superficial ones and the deeper ones of the midsection, commonly referred to as the "core."

Repeat the following circuit three times with two minutes of rest between circuits.

THE ZERO BELLY SWISS BALL WORKOUT

Exercise	Reps	Time
1. Wall Squat	15	-
2. Push-up	10	-
3. Balanced Sit	-	10 sec
4. Rollout	15	-
5. Hamstring Raise	10	-
6. Side Crunch	10	-
7. Wood Chop	10 each side	-
8. Alternate Arm/Leg Raise	10 each side	-
9. Rest		2 min

Repeat the circuit twice more, for a total of 3.

1. WALL SQUAT

Stand with your back to a wall and place a Swiss ball between your back and a wall at hip height, with your heels about two feet out from the wall and your arms hanging at your sides. Squat straight down, allowing the ball to roll up your back as you lower yourself. Stop when your thighs are parallel with the floor, then rise back up to complete one rep.

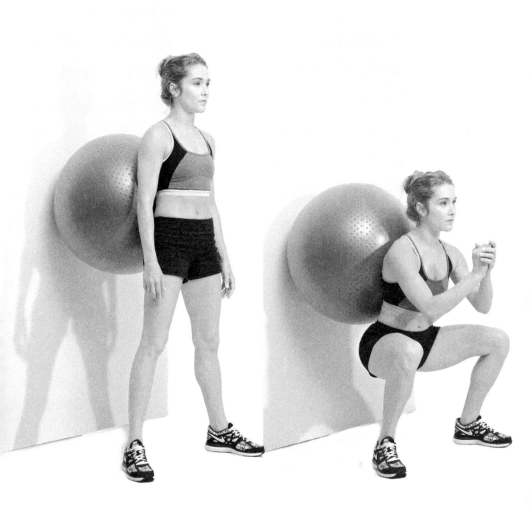

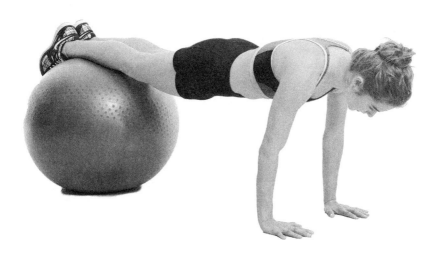

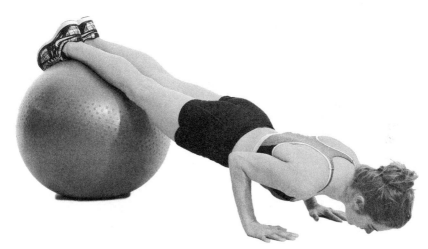

2. PUSH-UP

Perform as you would a normal push-up, except with either feet or shins placed on a Swiss ball. Feet on ball is the more difficult position; shin placement is easier. If stability is an issue, press the ball up against a wall, or in a corner.

3. BALANCED SIT

Sit on a Swiss ball with back straight and knees close together. With your hands either out to your sides or placed behind your head, raise both feet off the floor a couple of inches and attempt to hold for 10 seconds. To start you can press the ball against a wall for added stability.

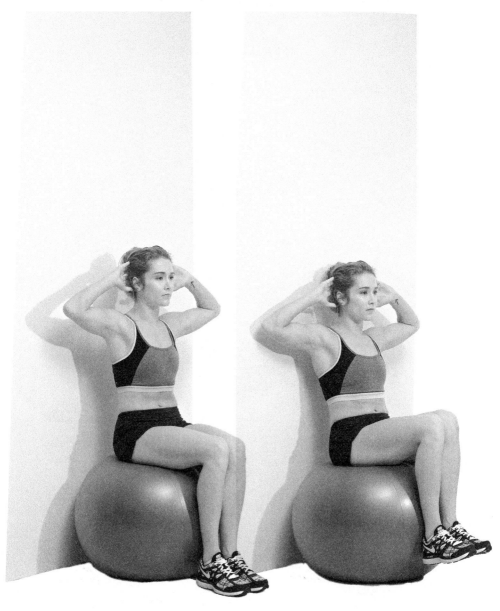

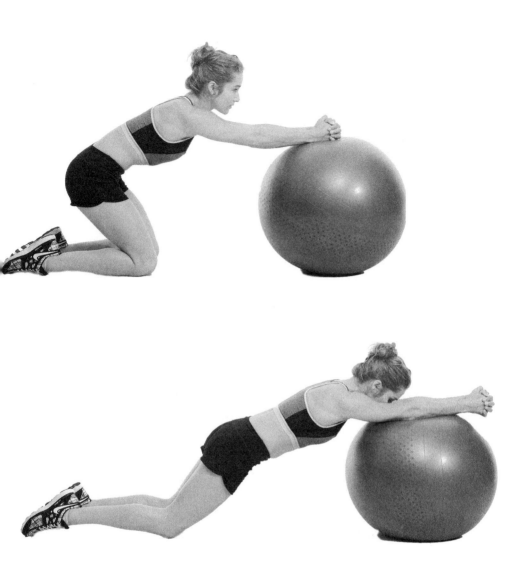

4. ROLLOUT

While resting on your knees, clasp your hands and place your forearms on the top of a Swiss ball. Extend your torso forward, rolling on your straightened arms, then pull back to the start position to complete one rep.

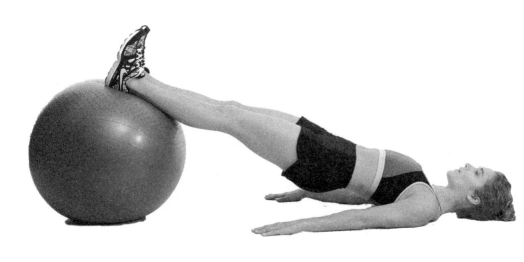

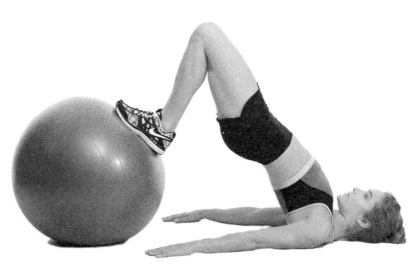

5. HAMSTRING RAISE

Lie on your back with a Swiss ball at your feet. Raise your legs up and place your heels and calves atop the ball. Now curl your lower legs back toward your glutes as you rise up on the ball, until the soles of your feet are on the ball and your hips are raised high. Slowly return to the start position to complete one rep.

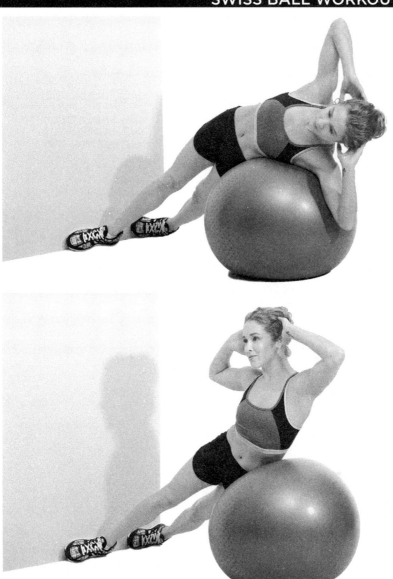

6. SIDE CRUNCH

Place a Swiss ball a couple of feet from a wall. Rest one hip against the ball while bracing your splayed feet in the crux of the wall and floor. Clasp your fingers behind your head and push the higher elbow toward the wall until your torso is nearly upright. Reverse the motion, getting a good stretch in your rib cage before pulling your torso back toward the wall.

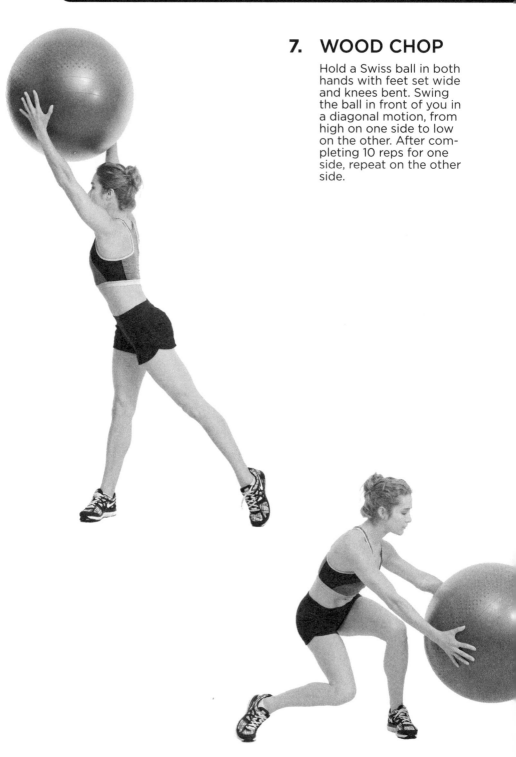

7. WOOD CHOP

Hold a Swiss ball in both hands with feet set wide and knees bent. Swing the ball in front of you in a diagonal motion, from high on one side to low on the other. After completing 10 reps for one side, repeat on the other side.

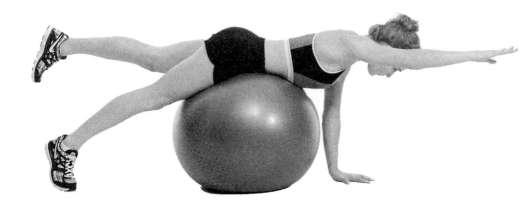

8. ALTERNATE ARM/LEG RAISE

Lie facedown on a Swiss ball with the ball directly under your abdomen. Keep the balls of both feet and/or hands on the floor. Raise your right arm and left leg until they're in line with your body and hold for a two count. Return to the starting position, then repeat with the alternate arm and leg.

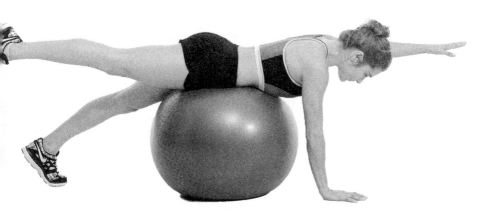

THE ZERO BELLY MEDICINE BALL WORKOUT

The medicine ball may well be the single oldest exercise tool know to man, with evidence of the ancient Greeks and Persians using sand-filled animal bladders some three thousand years ago. Fortunately, modern gyms have far less gross versions, but they're still essential equipment—because they're so effective at working the core.

There are two kinds of medicine balls: the kind made of soft material filled with sand or stuffed and weighted, and the newer rubber balls, some of which have a pair of molded handles. Either will work for the following workout, which should be performed four consecutive times with three minutes of rest between circuits.

THE ZERO BELLY MEDICINE BALL WORKOUT

Exercise	Reps	Time
1. Walking Lunge	20 steps	
2. Plank	-	20 sec
3. Floor Slam	10	
4. Alternating Push-up	5 each side	
5. V-Sit Rotation	10 each side	
6. Wall Sit		20 sec
7. Rest		3 min

Repeat the circuit 3 times (for a total of 4).

1. WALKING LUNGE

Hold a medicine ball with both hands at chest level. Take a large step forward and lower yourself until your rear knee brushes the floor. Your front lower leg should be perpendicular to the floor. Rise up as you take another step forward with your rear leg. Each step should be long, controlled, and deliberate.

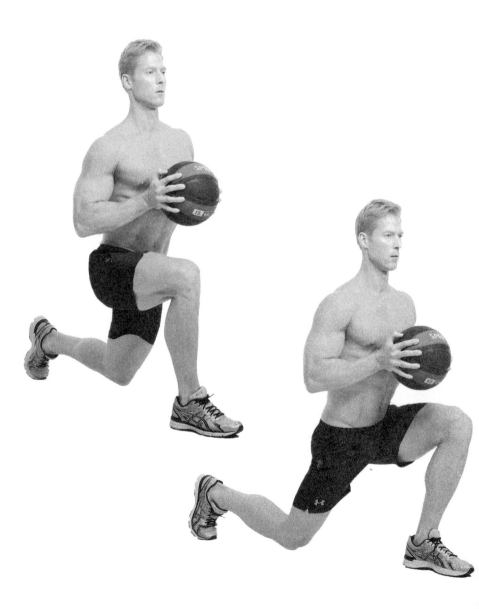

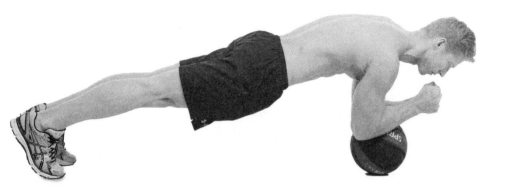

2. PLANK

Assume a standard plank position with your forearms resting atop a medicine ball. Make sure to keep your back straight and glutes engaged for 20 seconds.

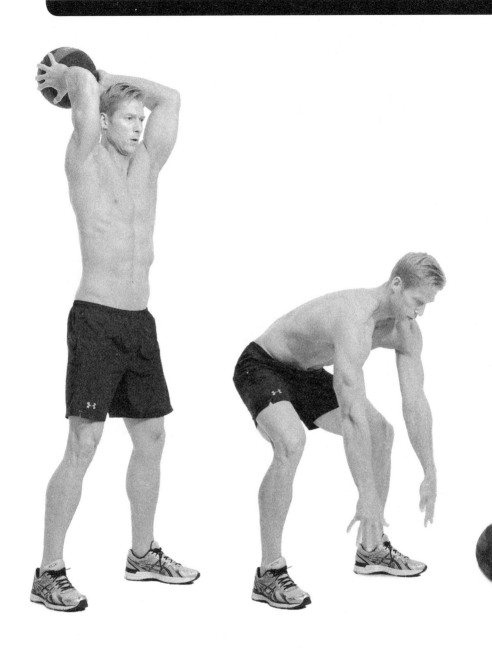

3. FLOOR SLAM

Lift a medicine ball overhead and then forcefully throw it down
to the floor a foot in front of you. Pick the ball back up and
repeat.

4. ALTERNATING PUSH-UP

Assume a push-up position, but with one hand atop a medicine ball. Perform a push-up. From the raised position, take the elevated hand off the ball and roll the ball over to your other hand, then move the elevated hand down to the floor. Do another push-up, this time with the opposite hand elevated.

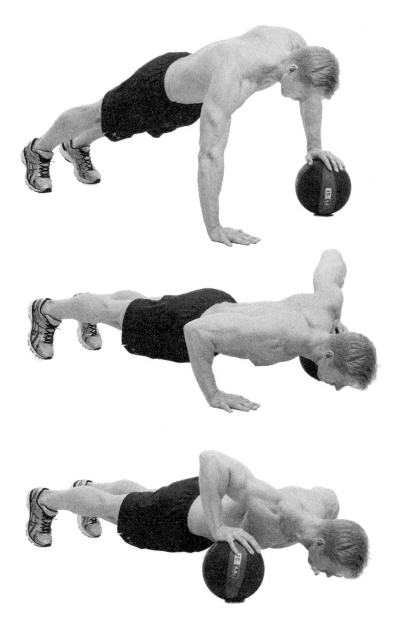

5. V-SIT ROTATION

Sit on the floor with your knees bent. Holding the medicine ball at chest level, lean back slightly as you lift your feet a few inches off the floor. Extend your arms in front of you and move the ball across your body, touching it to the floor to one side, then back across your body and touching it to the floor on the other side, at about hip level.

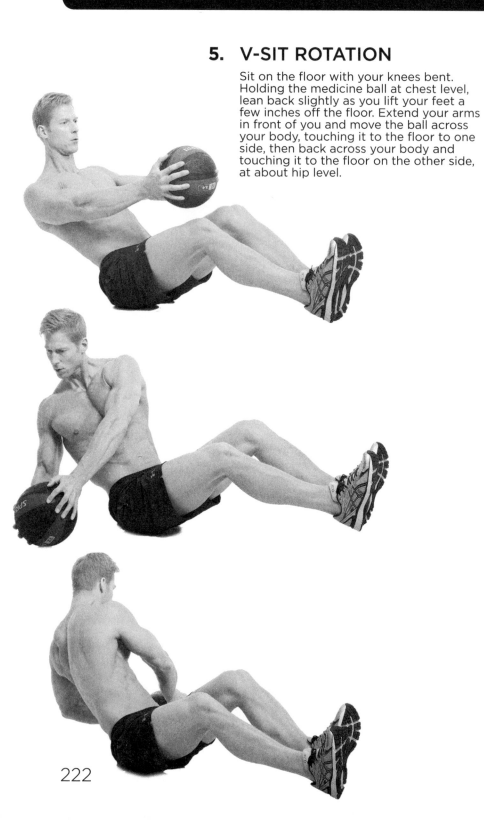

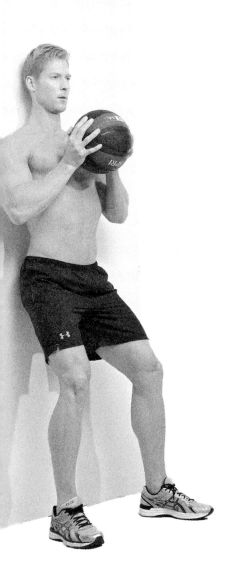

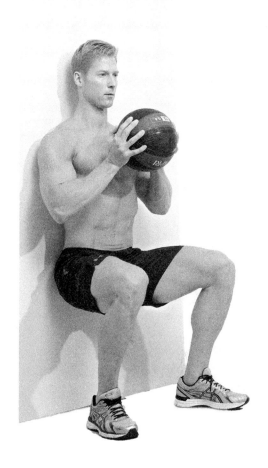

6. WALL SIT

Stand with your back facing a wall, with a distance of about a foot between the wall and your heels. Pick up a medicine ball and hold it at chest level. Lean back until your back is resting against the wall, then slide down the wall until your upper legs are parallel with the floor. Your lower legs should be perpendicular to the floor. Hold this position for 20 seconds.

CHAPTER TEN

ZERO BELLY IN SEVEN MINUTES A DAY

Superfast Core Workouts for Days When There's No Time to Work Out

Starting an exercise program is sort of like getting a jumbo jet off the ground. It takes an enormous amount of energy to get that lumbering beast down the runway and up into the air, but once you're moving forward with real speed, the actual flying isn't nearly as difficult.

But as with an airliner, once you stop, it's difficult to get going again. And that's why so many exercise programs fail. You get a couple of weeks or months of solid working out under your belt, and suddenly the kids get sick, or a work deadline looms, or the zombie apocalypse hits, and bam—you've missed two or four or six workouts in a row, and what's the point? You're back on the couch with Ben & Jerry.

That's where the Seven-Minute Abs Workouts come in. In between workout days or when you're on vacation, or when you simply can't raise enough bail money to get back to your routine, you can still get in a workout that will move you closer toward your ZERO BELLY goals. Most of these workouts require zero equipment, so you can do them almost anywhere, excuses be damned. And by adding strength to your core, you'll have even more impressive abs to show when your belly fat melts away.

Seven minutes, that's all I ask. Or rather, that's all you need to ask of yourself.

BEGINNER ABS WORKOUT

Perform the plank until you've held it for 90 seconds total—take as many sets as you need to get there. Between sets, rest the amount of time you held the plank for. So if you held it for 30 seconds in your first set, rest 30 seconds after that set. Go on to do the same with the side plank on both sides. As you get stronger, extend the length of time you hold each position.

1. PLANK

Reps: Hold for 90 sec

Rest: As long as you held the plank

Get into push-up position but with your upper body resting on your forearms. Brace your abs and hold your body in a straight line for as long as you can.

2. SIDE PLANK (left)

Reps: Hold for 60 sec total

Rest: As long as you held the side plank

Lie on your left side, resting your left forearm on the floor for support. Raise your hips up so that your body forms a straight line and brace your abs—your weight should be on your left fore-arm and the edge of your left foot.

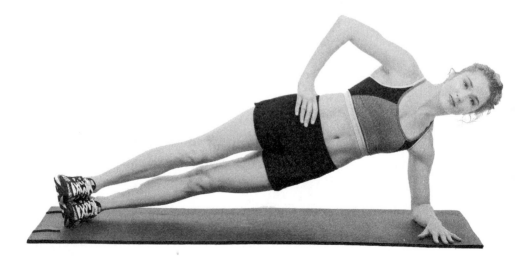

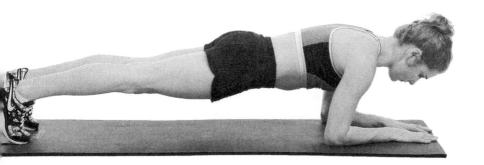

3. SIDE PLANK (right)

Reps: Hold for 60 sec total

Rest: As long as you held the side plank

Perform the side plank as described on opposite page, but on your right side.

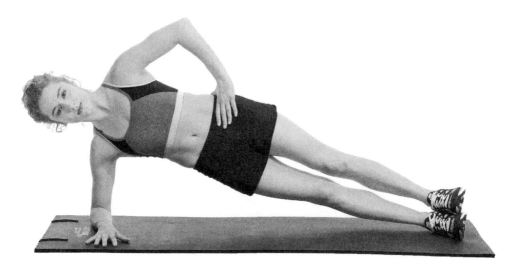

THE 360

In this routine you're going to rotate yourself 360 degrees on a lateral plane, starting with your back on the floor and ending in the same position. Along the way you will move clockwise through quarter turns, performing seven exercises total in a seven-minute span. You'll want to use an interval timer to alert you to each time you need to switch positions. By the end of minute seven you should be feeling the burn throughout your entire midsection, and will have set the stage for killer abs to come.

Exercises are to be performed in sequence with no rest between them.

Exercise	Time
1. Reverse Crunch	60 sec
2. Alternating Crunch	60 sec
3. Plank (right side)	60 sec
4. Plank	60 sec
5. Plank (left side)	60 sec
6. Reaching Crunch	60 sec
7. Bicycle Kicks	60 sec

1. REVERSE CRUNCH

Lie on your back with your hands placed palms down beside you and your legs held up perpendicular to the floor. Pulling with your abdominals, thrust your pelvis toward the ceiling and return to the start position in a controlled manner to complete one rep.

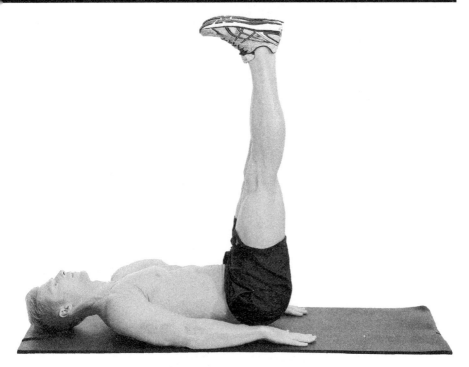

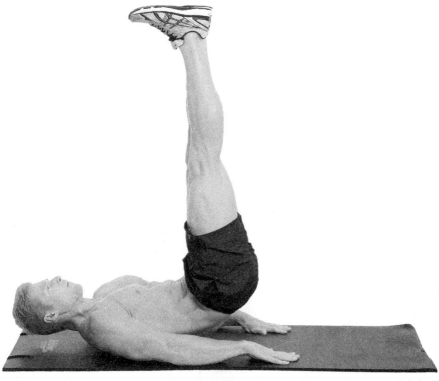

2. ALTERNATING CRUNCH

Lie on your back with your fingers clasped behind your head or your hands cupping your ears, and with your knees bent so that the soles of your feet are placed firmly on the floor. Curl your torso upward and rotate at the waist, trying to touch your right knee with your left elbow followed by your left knee with your right elbow. Continue alternating for 60 seconds.

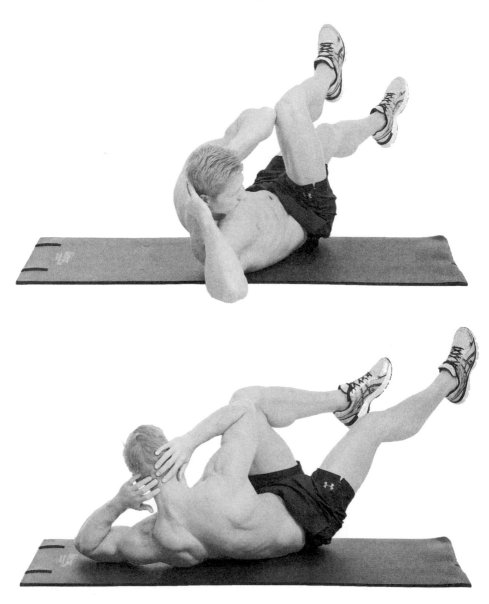

3. PLANK (right side)

Lie on the floor on your right side, then prop yourself up on your right elbow, making sure that your body is in a perfectly straight line.

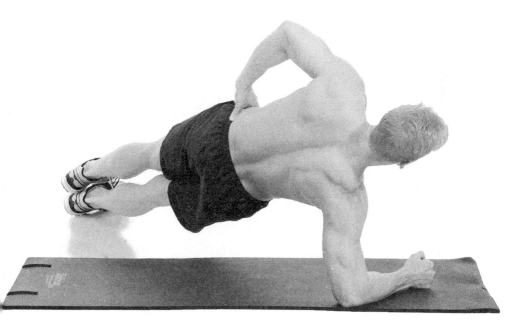

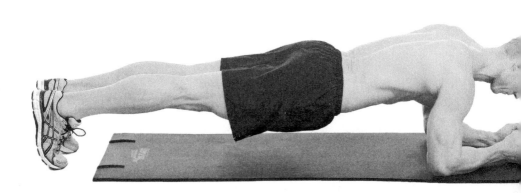

4. PLANK

Lie facedown on the floor, then prop yourself up on both elbows so that your arms form a 90-degree angle with your elbows directly under your shoulders. Keep your body straight from shoulders to feet. If the move is too difficult at first, take breaks in which you lower your knees to the floor for support.

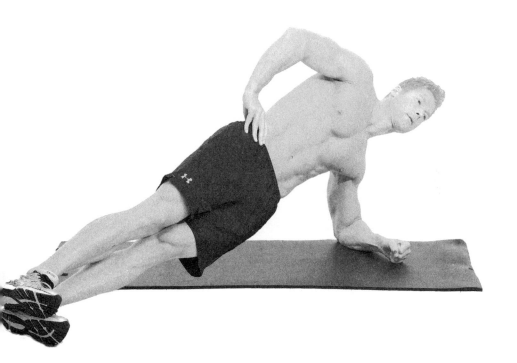

5. PLANK (left side)

Lie on the floor on your left side, then prop yourself up on your left elbow, making sure that your body is in a perfectly straight line. If the move is too difficult at first, lower the left knee to the floor for support.

6. REACHING CRUNCH

Lie on your back with your knees bent so that the soles of your feet are placed firmly on the floor. Hold your arms straight above you, so that they are perpendicular to the floor. Now reach as high as you can, imagining you're trying to touch the sky, then let your torso retract back into a supine position. Remember to roll up and back, rather than keeping a straight back.

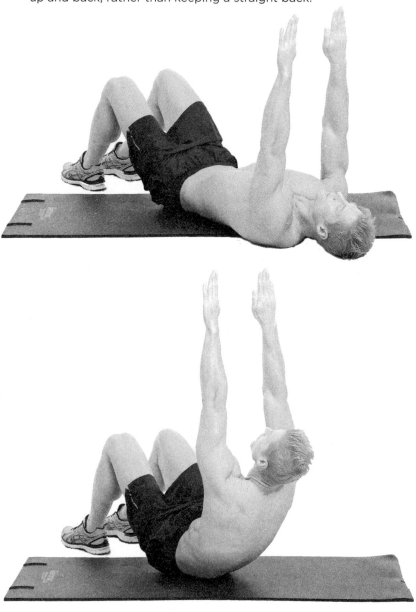

7. BICYCLE KICKS

Lie on your back with your fingers clasped behind your head or your hands cupping your ears, and with your hips and knees bent 90 degrees so your calves are parallel to the floor. Now pedal your feet in the air as if you were pedaling a bicycle, making small alternating circles.

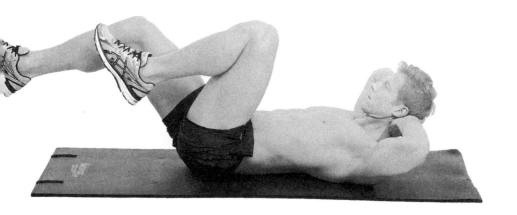

THE DYNAMIC DUO

Because it anchors your torso to your legs, your midsection receives a ton of work whenever you're moving dynamically. That's why track athletes and NFL running backs have such awesome abs. They didn't develop them by doing crunches and leg raises. It's the action of running itself that causes the abdominal muscles to contract forcefully as the legs and arms are pumped aggressively.

The following workout employs movements similar to those done by track athletes, resulting in a ballistic abs routine that will stealthily strengthen and develop your midsection as it burns calories, helping to further reveal the fruits of your labor. It consists of two "dynamic" exercises—running in place with high knees for thirty seconds, then burpees for thirty seconds—followed by 30 seconds of active rest in the form of a plank.

Exercise	Time
1. Run in Place (high knees)	30 sec
2. Burpee	30 sec
3. Plank	30 sec
REST: 20 sec	

Perform 4 circuits.

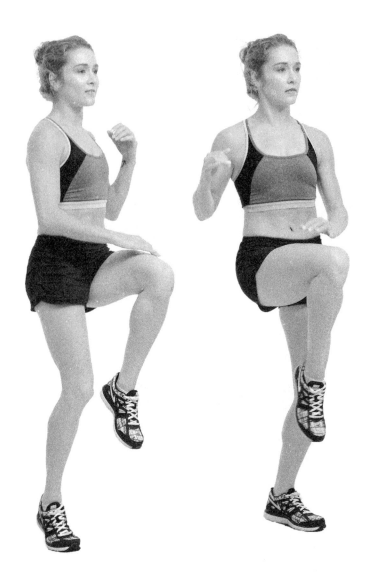

1. RUN IN PLACE (high knees)

When running in place, bring your knees at least up to hip level. To ensure they are high enough, you can start by holding your hands out in front of you at hip level. Aim to slap each knee against its opposite hand.

2. BURPEE

Stand with feet shoulder width apart. In one fluid motion,
first squat down and place your hands on the floor in front
of you, then thrust your feet straight back until you're in push-up
position. Bring your feet back to their original position,
then leap straight up, reaching high toward the ceiling to
complete one rep.

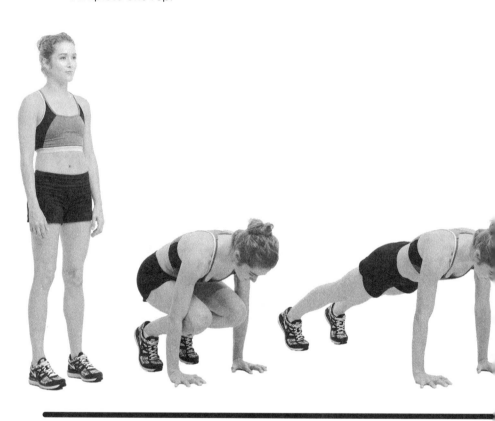

3. PLANK

Lie facedown on the floor, then prop yourself up on both elbows
so that your arms form a 90-degree angle with your elbows
directly under your shoulders. Keep your body straight from
shoulders to feet. If the move is too difficult at first, take breaks
in which you lower your knees to the floor for support.

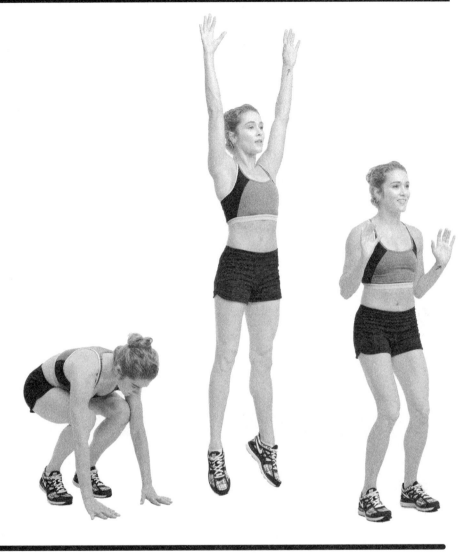

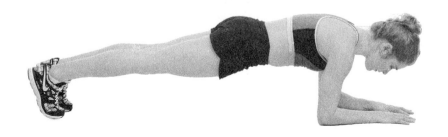

THE TIME WARP

Set a timer for seven minutes. Perform as many reps as you can for the first exercise, and then rest as needed. Go on to the next exercise and repeat. In the case of the plank, hold it as long as possible (instead of doing reps). Repeat the exercises in order until seven minutes are up. Count the reps you complete on each move and note your total at the end. Each time you repeat the workout, try to complete more total reps in the same amount of time.

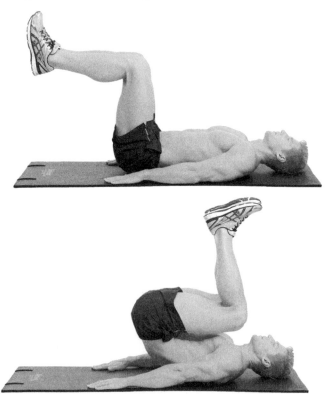

1. VERTICAL LEG CRUNCH

Lie on the floor on your back, with arms at your sides, palms facing down. Bend your hips and knees 90 degrees, so your calves are parallel to the floor. Brace your abs and roll your hips back toward you so they come up off the floor and your knees are at your chest. Roll your hips back to the floor.

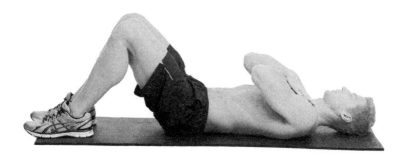

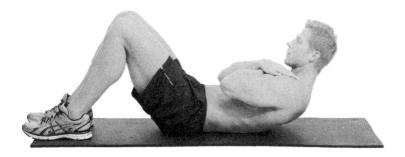

2. CRUNCH

Lie on the floor on your back, and bend your knees 90 degrees so your feet are flat on the floor. Cross your arms over your chest. Crunch your torso off the floor, coming up only until your shoulder blades are off the floor.

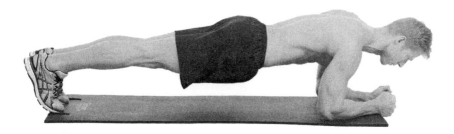

3. PLANK

Get into push-up position and then bend your elbows 90 degrees so your forearms lie flat on the floor. Brace your abs and hold your body in a straight line for as long as you can.

SEVEN MINUTES IN HELL

Use a timer and spend one minute performing each of these seven exercises. Do as many reps as you can in that time, resting as needed. Every time one minute is up, go on to the next exercise right away. For the plank and side planks, hold the positions for one minute each, or as long as you can. Each time you repeat the workout, try to perform more reps for each exercise.

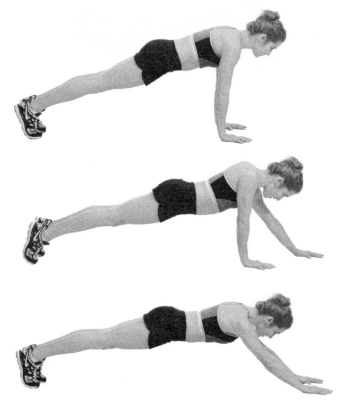

1. PUSH-UP WALKOUT

Get into push-up position, bracing your abs and holding your body straight. From there, walk your hands forward until you feel your lower back is about to sag. Walk your hands back and repeat.

2. LEG RAISE

Lie on the floor on your back and reach back to grab a chair, bench, or your partner's ankles for support. Keeping your legs straight, raise them up in the air until they're vertical. Lower them back down but stop an inch above the floor.

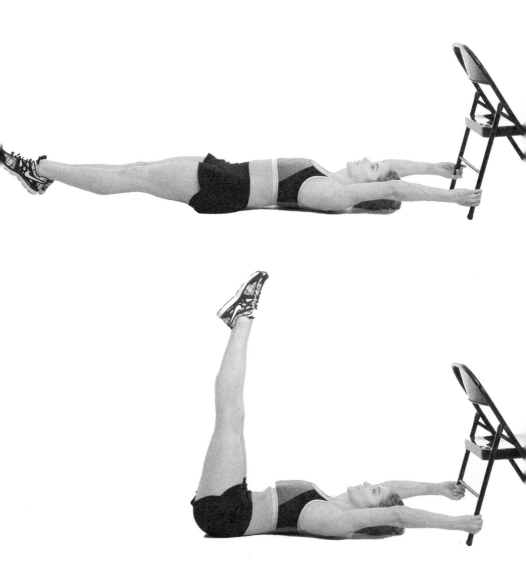

3. REACHING CRUNCH

Lie on the floor on your back and bend your knees 90 degrees so your feet are flat on the floor. Reach your arms overhead. Raise your torso until your shoulder blades are off the floor.

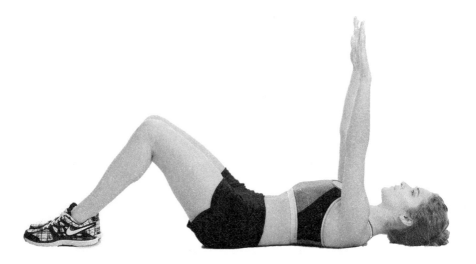

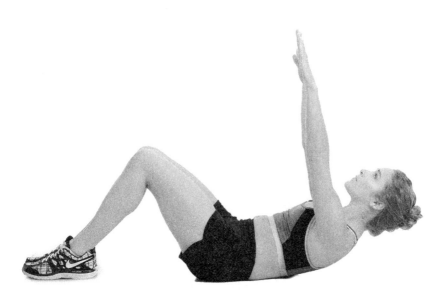

4. FLUTTER KICK

Lie on the floor on your back with your legs straight and your arms by your sides. Contract your abs and raise your legs off the floor a few inches. Rapidly kick your legs up and down in a scissor-like motion.

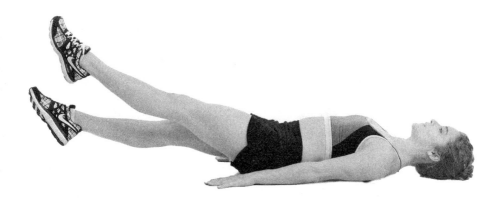

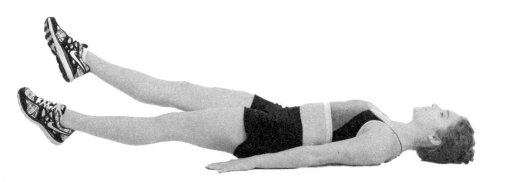

5. PLANK

Get into push-up position and then bend your elbows
90 degrees so your forearms lie flat on the floor. Brace your abs
and hold your body in a straight line for as long as you can.

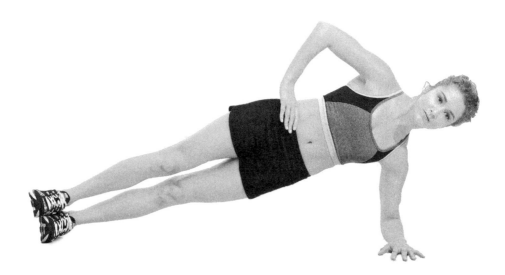

6. SIDE PLANK (left)

Lie on your left side, resting your left forearm on the floor for
support. Raise your hips up so that your body forms a straight
line and brace your abs—your weight should be on your left forearm and the edge of your left foot. Hold the position for as long
as you can.

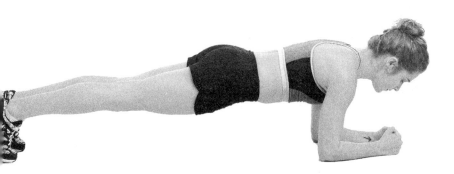

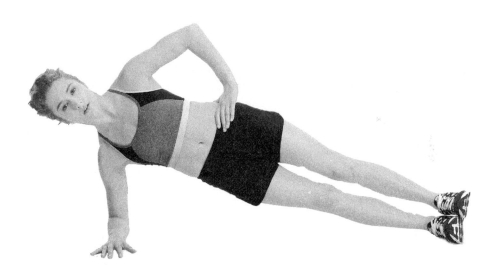

7. SIDE PLANK (right)

Perform the side plank as described above, but on your right side.

UP AND DOWN, SIDE TO SIDE

Alternate sets of the body saw and windshield wiper, resting 30 seconds after the body saw and 60 seconds after the windshield wiper. Perform 3 sets for each.

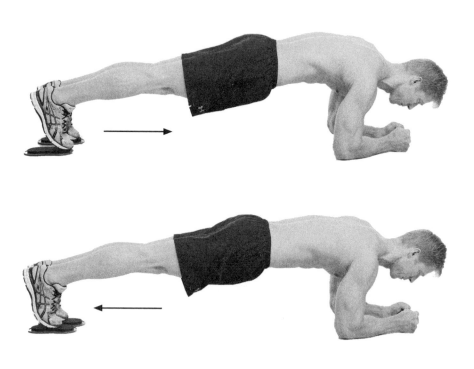

1. BODY SAW

Sets: 3 Reps 10–15

Rest: 30 sec

Get into push-up position and bend your elbows 90 degrees so your forearms are flat on the floor. Rest your feet on furniture sliders (available at any home improvement store), a towel (if you're on a waxed or smooth tiled floor), or paper plates. Keeping your abs braced, slide your body backward by pushing your forearms into the floor. Go as far as you can without your hips sagging. Then pull yourself forward as far as you can. That's one rep.

2. WINDSHIELD WIPER

Sets: 3 Reps: 8–10

Rest: 60 sec

Lie on your back on the floor with arms out 90 degrees to your sides. Raise your legs so they're straight and vertical. Twist your hips and lower your legs to your left side, but don't touch the floor. Repeat on the right side. That's one rep.

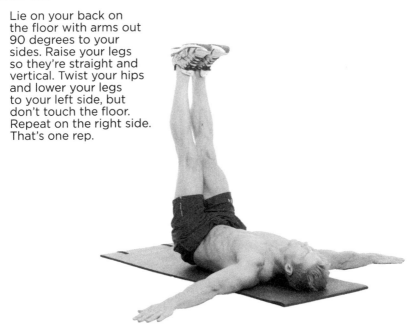

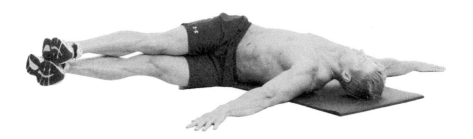

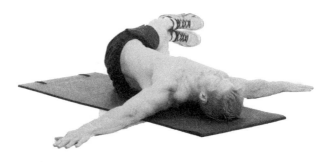

UNSTABLE GROUND

Perform the exercises as a circuit. Complete as many reps as you can for one move in thirty seconds, and then move on to the next exercise. Rest forty-five to sixty seconds after the circuit, and repeat for three total circuits.

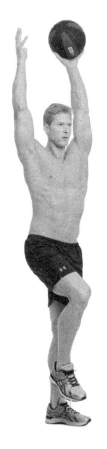 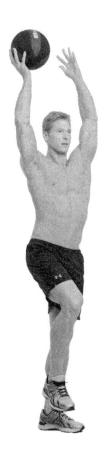

1. SINGLE-LEG BALL TOSS

Stand on one leg holding a light medicine ball, soccer ball, or other light ball overhead with the opposite side's hand. Brace your abs. Lightly and carefully pass the ball from hand to hand while maintaining your balance. Each pass is one rep. Continue balancing on the same leg until fatigued, then switch legs as needed.

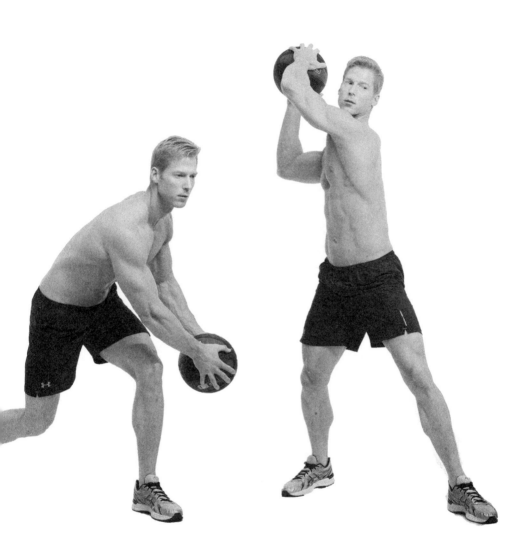

2. REVERSE CHOP

Get into a staggered stance and bend forward at the hips, holding a medicine ball to the outside of your front knee. Explosively swing the ball back and over the opposite shoulder (but don't let go). Your abs will have to work to slow your arms down. Perform reps for 15 seconds on one side and then switch legs and do 15 seconds on the other side.

3. RUSSIAN TWIST

Sit on the floor with knees bent and feet flat on the floor in front of you. Extend your arms, holding the ball in front of your chest. Explosively twist your body to one side as far as you can and then twist to the other side.

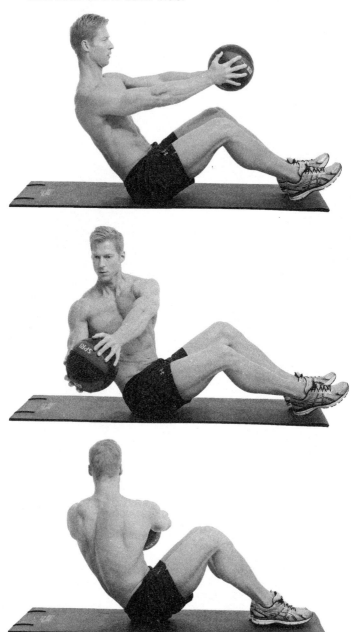

PLAYGROUND WORKOUT

Perform the exercises as a circuit, completing one set of each in turn and resting thirty seconds between each move. Repeat for seven minutes.

1. SWING SET FALLOUT

Reps: 8–10

Rest: 30 sec

> Stand behind a swing and grasp the seat with both hands, arms extended. Brace your abs and reach your arms forward so that your body lowers toward the ground; keep it in a straight line. Go until you feel you're about to lose tension in your abs, and then draw your arms back.

2. MONKEY BAR LEG RAISE

Reps: As many as possible

Rest: 30 sec

> Hang from monkey bars with hands at shoulder width. Contract your abs and raise your legs up to touch the bars. If that's too hard, bend your knees and raise them to your chest.

3. SWING SET SIDE PLANK

Reps: Hold as long as possible each side

Rest: 30 sec

> Lie on your left side, resting your left forearm on the ground for support. Rest your legs in the seat of a swing. Raise your hips up so that your body forms a straight line and brace your abs; your weight should be on your left forearm and the edge of your left foot. Hold for 30 seconds, then repeat with your right side.

Snaxercize!

Lower and regulate your blood sugar with short bursts of heart-pumping exercise.

Multiple, brief, snack-sized portions of exercise may control blood sugar better than a single, continuous workout, according to new research that adds to a growing body of evidence about the wisdom of spreading exercise throughout the day.

Scientists in New Zealand found that men and women with type 2 diabetes who engaged in three 10-minute exercise "hors d'oeuvres" before breakfast, lunch, and dinner saw lower postmeal blood sugar levels than they had in baseline testing. A single thirty-minute sweat session also lowered participants' blood glucose levels, but only among the exercise snackers were those effects visible throughout the day, not just after a meal, and they lingered for about twenty-four hours.

The longer ZERO BELLY workouts outlined in Chapter Ten are optimized to burn fat, build lean muscle, and strengthen your core, and they should constitute the majority of your exercise routine. But exercise snacking is great for days when you're strapped for time or when you've planned a Zero Guilt meal that's high in insulin-surging carbohydrates. Your ten-minute snack can consist of any type of physical activity, so long as it registers about a 9 on an exertion scale of 1–10. For some people, jogging at a moderate pace will be enough to work up a sweat, but as you become a fitter ZERO BELLY ninja, you'll have to increase the intensity of your snack attacks. Here's my favorite way to get your snack on.

10-MINUTE SNAXERCIZE CIRCUIT

1 minute jumping rope
1 minute jumping jacks
1 minute high knees
1 minute burpees
1 minute bodyweight squats
1 minute jumping rope
1 minute jumping jacks
1 minute high knees
1 minute burpees
1 minute bodyweight squats

CHAPTER ELEVEN

THE ZERO BELLY SEVEN-DAY CLEANSE

One Week to a Leaner, Cleaner, Healthier You

Before I tell you how you can weigh substantially less seven days from now, I'm going to let you in on a secret: I'm not really concerned about whether or not you weigh less seven days from now.

What matters to me is that you weigh less seven years from now. And seventeen years from now. And more. What I care about, and what I want you to focus on, is long-term success. I want you to enjoy a future filled with health, and the wealth and happiness that comes with it. I want you to reprogram your genetic destiny. I want you to be free from heart disease and diabetes. I want you to reduce your risk of Alzheimer's and cancer. I want you to slash your health care costs and boost your earning power. I want you to improve your sex life, lower your risk of injury, reverse digestive disorders, conquer autoimmune diseases, beat depression, and live a long, fulfilling, beautiful life for decades to come.

So no, I don't care what you weigh a week from now.

Life is a marathon, not a sprint, and you should never do anything in the short term that undermines your long-term chances of success.

Still . . . a short-term cleanse can be a smart long-term investment, especially since superfast results are a great way to motivate you toward a healthy future. So with that in mind, here's your seven-day plan for jump-starting a lifetime of weight loss.

THE SMART WAY TO CLEANSE

Near my hometown of Bethlehem, Pennsylvania, there's a beautiful trout stream called the Little Lehigh. For those enamored of the sport of fly-fishing, the stream holds one of the finest spots on the East Coast. But you can't take the trout home; it's strictly catch-and-release. You put the fish back, and return to perhaps catch it another day.

When it comes to weight-loss plans, I'm like one of those trout in the stream. When I see people promising that I can lose 10 pounds or more in just a week, I know—because I've been studying fitness and weight loss for more than twenty years—that such claims aren't reasonable. Yet I can't help but investigate. How are they doing this? What's the secret? Can that work for me? I rise to the bait, I'm easily hooked, and then I'm disappointed by reality and thrown back into the cold water. But I don't learn my lesson. I see another promise of rapid weight loss, and there I am, rising to the bait once again.

You're probably like that, too. It's human nature to get excited by quick-fix promises. Fact is, the only way you can lose massive amounts of weight in a very short period of time is to severely restrict calories. And that's something I'm not going to let you do. Severe calorie restriction might make you slim in seven days. But it will probably make you fat in seven years.

Here's why. One of the worst things you can do for your health, and your long-term weight-loss prospects, is to "go on a diet." When you decide to go on a diet, you're making the conscious decision that this is a temporary choice. You're going to go on it, but that means that one day—probably sooner than you expect—you're going to go off it. That's the concept of weight cycling (also known as yo-yo dieting), and it's extremely unhealthy. A 2014 study in the journal *Diabetes Care* found that a pattern of weight cycling—losing at least 5 pounds and then gaining it back within two years—resulted in as much as a 33 percent higher risk of diabetes and higher blood pressure. Another 2014 study called weight cycling "a widespread phenomenon in diabetes" and a contributing factor to depression as well.

That's in part because, when you restrict calories, you restrict nutrients. Your body goes into starvation mode, and it starts to look around for baggage to shed. And it would rather shed that cumbersome muscle—the stuff that's causing your metabolism to stay high and burn precious calories—than fat, which requires fewer calories to maintain. As a result, you lose weight on a crash diet, but much of it is muscle. Then, when you go off the diet—which you have to, because no severe calorie restriction diet is sustainable—your body is primed to gain the weight back, and more. With less muscle, your body's metabolism is set at a lower point. So eating even the exact same number of daily calories as you ate before causes you to gain more fat than you originally carried.

Then you go on another crash diet. And lose more muscle. And gain more weight. With less lean body tissue to store glycogen, your body is more susceptible to spikes in blood sugar, and your insulin receptors get burned out more quickly, setting you up for diabetes.

So don't do that.

I created ZERO BELLY to be a sustainable way of eating and living—one that you could follow for more than a few days, more than a few weeks or months. You can eat and live this way forever, and you can lose weight now and keep that weight off for good without restricting calories or harming your long-term health and weight.

So why did I create a seven-day cleanse? What makes it different from the ZERO BELLY lifestyle plan? And more important, what makes it different from those crash diets I warned you about?

The ZERO BELLY seven-day cleanse does three critical things. First, it reduces your calorie intake slightly, without radically altering the way you eat. There's no sudden, dramatic food restriction, just a mild cutting back on the way you're already eating, for a short period of time. Second, it incorporates short bouts of mild exercise to up your metabolic burn, without making you alter your lifestyle to include intense, hard-to-stick-to workouts. And third, it keeps your body fueled with clean, powerful, high-nutrient foods that have been proven to boost your health and lower your risk of disease while targeting unhealthy visceral fat.

You will lose weight, quickly and permanently, by following my core plan. But turbocharging your diet with a cleanse from time to time makes a lot of sense. Here's why:

Fast results help lead to long-term weight loss. Slow and steady is the best way to accomplish any personal goal, but sometimes the slow undermines the steady. A comprehensive review of studies conducted by researchers at the University of

Alabama, published in the *New England Journal of Medicine*, found that those who realized rapid results were more likely to stick to their weight-loss program over time than those who saw results come more slowly. In fact, those who lost the most weight within the first two weeks or so had the greatest total weight loss the following year. (The caveat: this applied only to healthy, high-nutrient diets, not gimmicks like weight-loss pills.) Which makes sense—we're human, after all, which means we're impatient and results-oriented. A second study from 2013 broke dieters into three groups: those who lost less than 5 percent of their body weight, those who lost between 5 and 10 percent, and a high-success group who lost 10 percent or greater. It found that the high-success group lost weight faster than the other groups; furthermore, this quick early weight loss made it more likely that participants would have maintained their weight loss as much as two years later. While ZERO BELLY is exactly the kind of high-nutrient plan that will give you rapid weight reduction, this seven-day cleanse can turbocharge those results—and a turbocharge at the start might improve your chances of long-term adherence to the plan.

Vacation happens. You're staying fit, focused, and disciplined and seeing great results, and then boom—you join the family on a cruise to Mexico and next thing you know you're at Señor Frog's, facedown in a pile of nachos and lime wedges. Getting back on the health horse is hard once you've fallen off, because you can start to feel like all your previous work was for naught. But it's critical, because falling back into a habit of eating poorly will set you up for the same lose-and-gain cycle I mentioned above. A quick cleanse after a holiday can get you back on track and prevent you from undermining your previous success.

Sometimes, taking charge feels good. Reunions come along from time to time. So do weddings, beach getaways, job interviews, big dates, and other "holy cow, I'd better get it in gear" moments. Taking control of our fitness and health at important junctures in life gives us a sense of accomplishment. Almost every culture and religion in history has promoted some kind of cleansing ritual, whether it's a period of fasting or a holiday in which certain foods are off-limits. Imposing a bit of self-discipline for a limited time can be a healthy thing for the mind and soul. A 2012 review of studies published in the *Journal of Sports Science* found that athletes who fasted for Ramadan, the Muslim religious observance, did not suffer any decrease in their athletic performance, as long as they kept their nutrient levels high and got adequate sleep. While you'll continue steady weight loss following ZERO BELLY, making a short-term sacrifice in order to realize a rapid leap forward can help keep your motivation intact.

Turbocharged results are within your grasp. What I love about this cleanse is that it doesn't require truly dramatic sacrifice. ZERO BELLY isn't a difficult program to follow by any means. So simply jump-starting it for seven days is an easy adjustment. The only serious change you'll need to make, besides giving up a daily snack, is in your morning routine.

HOW TO MAKE A CLEAN START

On the ZERO BELLY cleanse, you'll most likely see significant results within just the first seventy-two hours. Test panelists reported losing up to 3 inches off their waists in the first seven days of ZERO BELLY. Your results will be accelerated on this plan.

The ZERO BELLY cleanse is nothing more than a simple tweaking of the regular plan. It's just a little more intense, which is why I'm not recommending you make it your daily routine—it's a little hard to stick to for more than a week, so use it instead as a refresher course, the way you crammed during finals week to pass Applied Calculus. Here's what the plan looks like.

MEALS

Two ZERO BELLY drinks as meals (breakfast and lunch), one snack, a ZERO BELLY cleanse dinner, and no dessert. (Hey, it's only a week! I'll explain more about the dessert embargo below.) On the regular plan, you'd have three meals and two snacks, with one of those snacks being a drink. Here, I'm replacing both breakfast and lunch with drinks and eliminating one snack entirely, plus getting a little tough on you at dinnertime.

How Come? Since the drinks average about 300 calories each, this step alone will cut approximately 500 to 1,000 calories out of your daily intake, which may take several additional pounds off your body in just seven days. I've focused the ZERO BELLY cleanse on drinks because it's difficult to cut calories while maintaining the high levels of nutrients your body needs to remain healthy and support lean muscle tissue. The drinks pack such a nutritional punch that I know you'll be getting the vitamins, minerals, protein, and healthy fats you need. Remember to always ask the three ZERO BELLY questions before each meal or snack:

- **Where's my protein?**

- **Where's my fiber?**

- **Where's my healthy fat?**

CLEANSE DINNER

Okay, so you won't be dining at Waffle House this week. To make the cleanse work for you, you'll need to make your own dinners for the next seven days, or special-order off the menu of your favorite restaurant. Cleanse dinners consist of protein, vegetables, and healthy fats, but no grains or fruits. A little harsh, but again, it's only temporary.

How Come? Metabolism decreases up to 35 percent during sleep. That means that any extra carbs in your system at bedtime are more likely to get converted to glucose and then stored as fat. Grains and fruit are the two main sources of carbohydrates in the base ZERO BELLY plan, so I'm stripping them out for the next seven days.

ALCOHOL

None. Nada, nyet, nothing, no. Ixnay on the inksdray.

How Come? Alcohol is loaded with calories, to start with, so cutting down on booze is one of the fastest ways to get rid of empty calories. But alcohol is particularly bad for your weight because it's a toxin. Ingest a beer or a glass of wine and your body mobilizes to burn off the calories in that drink as quickly as possible, ignoring any other calories that might have come along with it. So whether it's wine and cheese or beer and wings, the drink gets metabolized while the body shoves a higher percentage of the accompanying food calories into fat cells.

CHEAT MEALS

None this week.

How Come? Dude, seriously. It's a cleanse.

WATER

Start each day by making a large pitcher of "spa water"—that's water filled with sliced whole lemons, oranges or grapefruits—and make a point of sipping your way through at least 8 glasses before bedtime. Citrus fruits are rich in the antioxidant d-limonene, a powerful compound found in the peel that stimulates liver enzymes to help flush toxins from the body and gives sluggish bowels a kick.

HOW TO BUILD A ZERO BELLY CLEANSE DINNER

1. Pick your protein (cooked any way you want, but with only 1 teaspoon of coconut or extra-virgin olive oil).

- **5 ounces chicken breast** (skinless)
- **5 ounces lean ground turkey**
  (at least 93 percent lean)
- **5 ounces lean ground beef**
  (at least 90 percent lean, preferably grass-fed)
- **5 ounces lean steak**
  (sirloin or anything labeled round, preferably grass-fed)
- **5 ounces fish** (preferably wild-caught)
- **2 eggs plus 1 or 2 egg whites**

2. Steam, stir-fry, or build a salad with some combination of these vegetables, and feel free to indulge in 2 or 3 heaping cups. (Note that cruciferous vegetables such as cabbage, broccoli, and cauliflower are not on the list, as they can cause bloating. While you may enjoy them as part of the main diet, I'm again stripping them out here for accelerated results.)

- **Spinach**
- **Romaine or other lettuce**
- **Asparagus**
- **Grape tomatoes**
- **Carrots**
- **Bell peppers**
- **Mushrooms**
- **Zucchini or squash**
- **Herbs and spices**

Top salads with 1 tablespoon Zero Belly Vinaigrette (page 102).

3. Add a fat (but only if no fat exists in the recipe already)

- **¼ avocado**
- **1 tablespoon nuts or seeds**
- **1 tablespoon of your favorite nut butter**

How Come? On this cleanse, you're going to be eating a little less food, which means you're going to be getting a little less water—much of the water we ingest actually comes from our food. Plus, you're going to be exercising just a little more, which means you're going to be giving off more water in the form of exhalation and maybe a little sweat, too. That means you're going to need more water than you normally drink. In addition, water will keep you full, helping to stanch cravings. Often what we interpret as hunger is actually thirst.

FOOD AND EXERCISE PLAN

	MONDAY	TUESDAY	WEDNESDAY
WORKOUT	Circuit	Cardio	Circuit
BREAKFAST	Vanilla Milkshake	The Peanut Butter Cup	Mango Muscle-Up
LUNCH	Blueberry Dazzler	Strawberry Banana	Vanilla Milkshake
SNACK	1 apple & 2 Tbsp nut butter	1 cup berries & 2 Tbsp almonds	1 cup raw vegetable sticks & 2 Tbsp nut butter
DINNER	Grilled Chicken & Steamed Veggies & Avocado	Poached Eggs & Grilled Veggies & 2 Tbsp Peanut Butter	Grilled Salmon & Mixed Greens

EXERCISE

Every other day, you'll follow one of the ZERO BELLY workouts. But there's more: in addition to your regular workout, you'll start each of the next seven mornings with a thirty-minute aerobic workout *before breakfast* to jump-start your metabolism.

How Come? More and more studies have shown that "fasted" exercise—meaning a workout before breakfast—is a more effective fat-burner than exercise later in the day. The key is to do a

THURSDAY	FRIDAY	SATURDAY	SUNDAY
Cardio	Circuit	Cardio	Circuit
Vanilla Milkshake	Strawberry Banana	Blueberry Dazzler	The Peanut Butter Cup
The Peanut Butter Cup	Mango Muscle-Up	Vanilla Milkshake	Strawberry Banana
1 apple & 2 Tbsp nut butter	1 cup berries & 2 Tbsp almonds	1 cup raw vegetable sticks & 2 Tbsp nut butter	1 apple & 2 Tbsp nut butter
Turkey (grilled as burger) with Lettuce, Tomato & Avocado	Grilled Chicken & Mixed Greens & 2 Tbsp walnuts	Pan Seared Halibut & Stir Fried Veggies & 2 Tbsp cashews	Grilled Flank Steak & Mixed Greens & Avocado

light workout before you eat anything—no latte, no Gatorade, no Luna bar or apple or "something small." Once you eat, you give your body a boost of glycogen—the energy that powers your day. So now when you go to exercise, you need to burn off that glycogen. But work out before you eat, and your burn will come primarily from fat. A study from Northumbria University found that people burn up to 20 percent more body fat by exercising in the morning on an empty stomach.

Here's the reason for that phenomenon. Your body has two sources of stored calories—glycogen, which is stored in the muscles and liver, and fat, which is stored you-know-where. The liver and muscles can hold about 1,500 or so calories' worth of glycogen.

Fortunately, your body is a pretty efficient calorie-burning machine. Even just lying around, sleeping, watching TV, and snacking normally, the average 185-pound man smokes through a little more than 1,900 calories over the course of twenty-four hours. So if you stop eating at 7:00 p.m., collapse on the couch, then wake up at 7:00 a.m., you've already burned through 950 calories just lying there. But chances are you did at least a few other things—washed the dishes, played with the dog, threw darts down in the rec room—before going to sleep. So let's say that 950 is more like 1,200 or so. As a result, when you wake up you have very few calories stored as glycogen.

Now what happens when you start to exercise without eating? You quickly zip through your glycogen stores and tap into fat—that's why so many of your "fasted" calories come from fat. But this plan is most effective if you stop eating early enough the night before. (That means no dessert for the week of the cleanse.)

What kind of exercise should you do? It's not that important. A 150-pound woman will burn about 250 calories in a half hour of most moderate aerobic exercise—biking, light jogging, tennis, swimming, or following along with an aerobics class. That may not sound like much, but the calories you do burn are calories that count.

Exercising before your morning meal is also one of the best

ways to erase the damage caused by dietary mistakes. That makes this plan perfect if you've just overdone it during a holiday. In a 2010 study published in the *Journal of Physiology*, researchers fed a group of active men an unhealthy diet composed of 50 percent fat and 30 percent more calories than they normally consumed. (Blecch!) They then divided the men into three subgroups: one group wasn't allowed to exercise at all, another group exercised four times a week after eating breakfast, and the third group exercised four times a week before eating their first meal of the day. The no-exercise group gained 6 pounds, developed insulin resistance (the precursor to diabetes), and began storing fat in their muscle cells. The group that exercised after eating breakfast gained about 3 pounds and also showed signs of insulin resistance and greater fat storage. But the participants who exercised before eating their first meal gained almost no weight and showed zero signs of insulin resistance.

That's right: as long as they exercised before breakfast, they could eat all they wanted and had no weight gain.

DESSERT

Nope, none of that either. In fact, I don't want you to eat anything after 7:00 p.m. if possible.

How Come? If you end your eating by 7:00 p.m., you'll set yourself up to begin burning fat first thing in the morning. Not just burning calories—burning fat.

As you go through the ZERO BELLY cleanse, you'll experience a sense of control over your diet, your body, and your health. One of the reasons so many religions and cultures impose periods of cleansing is that they help to bring discipline and focus to your life. And in this case, the focus is going to be on you—and how terrific you look.

5 TEAS THAT SPEED WEIGHT LOSS

What if I told you there was a soothing and tasty, calorie- and additive-free elixir on the market with the ability to cleanse away dietary sins, speed up weight loss, and even prevent disease? Yes! It's true: Tea may be the healthiest drink on the planet.

In fact, people have been enjoying soothing tea and it's impressive benefits for *thousands* of years. One legend dates the discovery of tea to 2737 B.C. by the emperor of China. Fast-forward some 4,700 years and researchers circa 2014 now have clinical studies that prove tea can help with cancer, heart disease, and diabetes; encourage weight loss; lower cholesterol; and bring about mental alertness.

Rich in antioxidants and relatively low in caffeine (a cup of coffee has about 100 mg where a cup of green tea has a mere 25 mg), there are dozens of teas available that you can sip safely throughout the day. Stick to 3–4 cups (or tea bags) of tea per day during your ZERO BELLY cleanse, and choose brewed teas over bottled to avoid extra calories and sweeteners. Decaffeinated varieties are great to have on hand for a soothing bedtime treat.

Here's a primer on the best teas for a trimmer tummy.

GREEN TEA

Benefit: Helps burn more calories at the gym

Brands to love:
Lipton
Yogi

Forget shelling out cash on trendy preworkout supplements! The secret supernutrients in green tea are called catechins, belly-fat crusaders that blast adipose tissue by revving the metabolism, increasing the release of fat from fat cells (particularly in the belly), and then speeding up the liver's fat-burning capacity.

OOLONG TEA

Benefit:
Boosts fat metabolism

Brands to love:
Bigelow
Stash

Oolong, a Chinese name for black dragon, is a semi-oxidized tea with a light, floral taste. Like green tea it's also packed with catechins, which help to promote weight loss by boosting your body's ability to metabolize lipids (fat). A study in the *Chinese Journal of Integrative Medicine* found that participants who regularly sipped on oolong tea lost six pounds over the course of six weeks.

MINT TEA

Benefit:
Wards off the munchies

Brands to love:
Tazo
Teavana
Celestial Seasonings
Sleepytime (an essential night-time treat!)

Fill a big tea cup with soothing peppermint tea, and sniff yourself skinny! One study published in the *Journal of Neurological and Orthopaedic Medicine* found that people who sniffed peppermint every two hours lost an average of 5 pounds a month! Consider also adding a few drops of peppermint oil to your pillow or burning a minty candle to fill the room with slimming smells.

WHITE TEA

Benefit: Blocks new fat cells from forming

Brands to love:
Twinings
The Republic of Tea

White tea is dried naturally, often in sunlight, making it the least processed and richest source of antioxidants among teas (as much as three times as many polyphenols as green tea!). A study published in the journal *Nutrition and Metabolism* showed that white tea can simultaneously boost lipolysis (the breakdown of fat) and block adipogenesis (the formation of fat cells) due to high levels of ingredients thought to be active on human fat cells, such as methylxanthines (like caffeine) and epigallocatechin-3-gallate (EGCG).

RED TEA

Benefit: Regulates hunger signals

Brands to love:
Celestial Seasonings
Harney & Sons

Rooibos tea is made from the leaves of the "red bush" plant, grown exclusively in the small Cederberg region of South Africa, near Cape Town; so you can feel very glam and worldly as you sip your bright red brew. What makes rooibos tea particularly good for your belly are powerful compounds, namely the flavanoid Aspalathin, that research shows can prevent stress hormone imbalances intricately linked to clinical conditions like hypertension, metabolic syndrome, cardiovascular disease, insulin resistance, and type 2 diabetes. Think: Red Rooibos for R&R!

THE HEALTHIEST FOODS ON THE PLANET

Maximize Your Nutritional Intake with This At-a-Glance Guide to All Your Favorite Foods

If you've made it all the way to this page, then you're clearly sold on the benefits of the **ZERO BELLY** way of eating and committed to changing your life through smart, groundbreaking nutrition. Either that, or you're just reading this book backwards.

- = Nutritional content not available

Food	Calories	Protein	Fiber	Carbohydrate	Total Fat	Saturated Fat	Monounsaturated	Polyunsaturated	Omega 3s (mg)	Sodium (mg)
Almond butter (1 tbsp)										
	101	2	1	3	9.5	0.9	6.1	2	67.7	1.8
Almond milk, unsweetened (8 oz)										
	40	1	1	2	3	0	~	~	~	180
Almonds (1 oz)										
	161	6	3	6	13.8	1	8.6	3.4	1.7	0.3
Apple										
	65	0	3	17	0	0	0	0	11.2	1.3
Apricot										
	17	0	1	4	0	0	0	0	0	0.4
Artichoke										
	60	4	7	13	0	0	0	0	21.8	120
Asparagus (1 spear)										
	3	0	0	1	0	0	0	0	1.6	0.3
Avocado (1 fruit)										
	227	3	9	12	21	2.9	13.3	2.5	150	10.9
Bacon (3 slices)										
	128	13	0	0	13	4.2	5.6	1.4	59.6	233
Bagel (4-inch)										
	229	9	2	45	1	0.3	0.5	0.6	57	399
Banana										
	105	1	3	27	0.4	0	0	0	31.9	1.2

Either way, finding exactly the best source for your daily sustenance can be a challenge—even at the salad bar, when you're paying by the pound, it's hard to know whether to splurge for the carrots or the cauliflower. And then there's the complicated stuff, from egg sandwiches to coffee cake. How good is the good stuff—and how much of a splurge is the bad stuff? Here, from aardvark chops to zebra loin—okay, not really, but it is an A-to-Z guide—is your quick and handy cheat sheet to the foodstuffs that cross your path every day.

Vitamin A (mcg)	Vitamin B1 (mg)	Vitamin B6 (mg)	Folate (mcg)	Vitamin C (mg)	Vitamin E (mg)	Calcium (mg)	Magnesium (mg)	Potassium (mg)	Selenium (mcg)	Zinc (mg)
0	0	0	10.4	0.1	~	43.2	0.4	121	~	0.5
500	~	~	~	0	10	200	16	~	~	~
0	0.05	0.03	11	0	6	71	86	180	0	1
8	0.02	0.06	4	6	0.25	8	7	148	0	0.06
67	0.01	0.02	3	3.5	0.3	5	3.5	90	0.03	0.07
0	0.1	0.15	87	15	0.24	56	77	474	0.26	0.6
12	0.02	0.01	8	1	0.18	4	2	32	0.37	0.1
122	0.2	0.6	124	16	3	22	78	1,204	0.8	0.84
0	0.08	0.07	0.4	0	0.06	2	6	107	12	0.7
0	0.15	0.05	20	0	0.04	16	26	90	28	1
7	0.04	0.4	24	10	0.12	6	32	422	1	0.2

Food	Calories	Protein	Fiber	Carbohydrate	Total Fat	Saturated Fat	Monounsaturated	Polyunsaturated	Omega 3s (mg)	Sodium (mg)
Beans, baked (1 cup cooked)										
	283	4	11	53	3.6	1.2	1.3	1	35.4	845
Beans, black (1 cup cooked)										
	227	15	15	41	0.9	0.2	0.1	0.4	181	1.7
Beans, kidney (1 cup cooked)										
	219	16	16	40	0.2	0	0	0.1	56.6	7.1
Beans, lima (1/2 cup cooked)										
	108	7	7	19	0.4	0.1	0	0.2	47	1.9
Beans, navy (1 cup cooked)										
	255	15	19	48	1.1	0.2	0.3	0.9	322	0
Beans, pinto (1 cup cooked)										
	245	15	15	45	1.1	0.2	0.2	0.4	234	1.7
Beans, refried (1 cup cooked)										
	201	13	11	34	2.1	0.3	0.5	1.1	424	1,040
Beef, ground lean (3 oz)										
	279	12	0	0	25.2	9.6	11.1	0.6	52.2	56.4
Beer (12 oz)										
	153	2	0	13	0	0	0	0	0	14.2
Beets (1/2 cup)										
	29	1	2	6	0	0	0	0	0	3.4
Blueberries (1 cup)										
	84	1	4	21	0.5	0	0.1	0.2	85.8	1.5
Bran, wheat (1 cup)										
	125	9	25	37	2.5	0.4	0.4	1.3	96.9	1.2
Bread, rye (1 slice)										
	83	3	2	15	1.1	0.2	0.4	0.3	19.2	211
Bread, white (1 slice)										
	120	3	1	23	1.5	0.3	0.3	0.6	62.6	306
Bread, whole-grain (1 slice)										
	69	3	2	11	1.1	0.2	0.2	0.5	53.3	109
Breakfast sandwich, fast-food (bacon, egg, and cheese)										
	432	19	1	32	27	11.7	7.9	3.7	0	1,225
Broccoli (1 cup)										
	31	3	2	6	0.3	0	0	0	19.1	30
Brussels sprouts (1/2 cup)										
	38	3	3	8	0.3	0.1	0	0.1	87.1	22
Cake, coffee (1 piece)										
	238	4	1	27	13.3	3.3	7.4	1.8	88.9	200

Vitamin A (mcg)	Vitamin B₁ (mg)	Vitamin B₆ (mg)	Folate (mcg)	Vitamin C (mg)	Vitamin E (mg)	Calcium (mg)	Magnesium (mg)	Potassium (mg)	Selenium (mcg)	Zinc (mg)
13	0.4	0.34	61	8	1.35	127	81	752	12	4
1	0.4	0.12	256	0	0.14	46	120	610	2	1.9
0	0.28	0.21	230	2	0.05	62	74	717	2	1.8
32	0.12	0.16	22	9	0.12	27	63	485	1.7	0.7
0.36	0.4	0.3	255	1.64	0.73	127	107	670	11	1.9
0	0.17	0.16	294	1.37	1.61	72	70	495	19	1.7
0	0.07	0.36	28	0	1.74	161	113	1,004	2.3	2.5
0	0.06	0.24	7	0	0.15	7	19	265	0	4
0	0.02	0.18	21	0	0	18	21	89	2.5	0.04
0	0.02	0.05	74	3	0.03	11	16	221	0.5	0.24
17	0.11	0.15	17	28	1.65	17	17	223	0.3	0.5
0	0.14	0.35	14	0	0.54	26	220	426	28	3
0.26	0.14	0.02	35	0.13	0.11	23	13	53	10	0.36
0	0.11	0.02	28	0	0.06	38	6	25	4.3	0.2
0	0.11	0.1	30	0.08	0.09	24	14	53	9	0.3
0	0.53	0.16	73	2	0.6	160	25	211	36	2
213	0.05	0.11	50	66	0.33	34	18	230	2	0.3
60	0.08	0.14	47	48	0.34	28	16	247	1.17	0.26
20	0.1	0.03	27	0.11	0.11	76	10	63	9	0.25

Food	Calories	Protein	Fiber	Carbohydrate	Total Fat	Saturated Fat	Monounsaturated	Polyunsaturated	Omega 3s (mg)	Sodium (mg)
Cake, frosted (1 piece)										
	243	2	1	35	11.1	3	6.1	1.4	68.5	216
Canadian bacon (2 slices)										
	89	12	0	1	4	1.3	1.8	0.4	51.3	803
Candy, non-chocolate (1 package)										
	250	0	0	56	2.7	2.6	0	0	0	9.3
Cantaloupe (1 medium wedge)										
	23	1	1	6	0.1	0	0	0.1	31.7	11
Carrot (1)										
	25	1	2	6	0.1	0	0	0.1	1.2	42.1
Cashews (1 oz)										
	155	5	1	9	12.3	2.2	6.7	2.2	17.4	3.4
Cauliflower (1 cup)										
	25	2	3	5	0.1	0	0	0	37	30
Celery (1 cup, strips)										
	16	1	2	3	0.2	0	0	0.1	0	80.8
Cereal, whole-grain, with raisins										
	187	6	7	45	1.5	0.2	0.3	0.6	47.2	289
Cheddar cheese (1 slice)										
	113	7	0	0	9.3	5.9	2.6	0.3	102	174
Chef's salad with no dressing (½ cups)										
	210	20	3	9	9	4.5	~	~	~	960
Cherries, sweet, raw (1 cup)										
	87	1	3	22	0.3	0.1	0.1	0.1	35.9	0
Cherries, tart (1 cup)										
	88	2	3	22	0.2	0.1	0.1	0.1	36.6	17.1
Chia seeds (1 oz)										
	137	4	11	12	8.6	0.9	0.6	6.5	4,915	5.3
Chicken, skinless (½ breast)										
	130	27	0	0	1.5	0.4	0.4	0.3	47.2	76.7
Chickpeas (1 cup cooked)										
	269	15	12	45	4.2	0.4	1	1.9	70.5	11.5
Chili with beans (1 cup)										
	287	15	11	30	14.1	6	6	0.9	392	1,336
Chips, potato, lite (1 oz)										
	132	2	2	19	5.8	1.2	1.3	3.1	53.2	138
Chocolate, dark (1 oz)										
	163	2	2	15	10.7	6.2	3.2	0.3	24.6	2.8

Vitamin A (mcg)	Vitamin B1 (mg)	Vitamin B6 (mg)	Folate (mcg)	Vitamin C (mg)	Vitamin E (mg)	Calcium (mg)	Magnesium (mg)	Potassium (mg)	Selenium (mcg)	Zinc (mg)
10	0.01	0.02	7	0.04	0	18	14	84	1.4	0.3
0	0.4	0.2	2	0	0.16	5	10	181	11	0.8
0	0	0	0	0	0	0	0	0	0	0
345	0.04	0.07	21	37	0.05	9	12	272	0.4	0.18
734	0.04	0.08	12	4	0.4	20	7	195	0.06	0.15
0	0.1	0.1	7	0.1	0.3	10.4	81.8	185	5.6	1.6
2	0.06	0.22	57	46	0.08	22	15	303	0.6	0.3
55	0.03	0.1	45	4	0.33	50	14	322	0.5	0.16
3	0.16	0.1	22	0.55	0.4	33	70	207	10	1
75	.01	.02	5	0	.08	204	8	28	4	.9
146	.4	.4	101	16	0	235	49	401	37	3
30	.07	.05	5.8	10	.2	21	16	325	.9	.09
1,840	0	0.1	19.5	5.1	0.6	26.8	14.6	239	0	0.2
~	~	~	~	~	~	177	~	44.8	~	1
4	.04	.32	2	.71	.08	6.5	16	150	11	.5
4	.19	.22	282	2	.6	80	79	477	6	2.5
87	.12	.3	59	4	1.46	120	115	934	3	5
0	0.5	0.22	8	3.4	0.62	10	18	285	2	0.17
14	0	0	~	~	~	17.4	49.3	159	2.4	0.7

Food	Calories	Protein	Fiber	Carbohydrate	Total Fat	Saturated Fat	Monounsaturated	Polyunsaturated	Omega 3s (mg)	Sodium (mg)
Chocolate, milk (1.55 oz [standard bar])										
	235	3	1	26	13	8.1	3.2	0.6	53.7	34.8
Cinnamon bun (1)										
	260	3	1	28	16	4	~	~	~	125
Citrus juice (12 oz)										
	112	0	0	28	0	0	0	0	-	25
Clams, breaded and fried (³⁄₄ cup)										
	172	12	0	9	9.5	2.3	3.9	2.4	294	309
Coconut milk, light (4 oz)										
	125	1	0	6	11	6	~	~	~	20
Coconut oil (1 tbsp)										
	116	0	0	0	13.5	11.7	0.8	0.2	~	0
Coffee (1 cup)										
	2	0	0	0	0	0	0	0	~	4.7
Collards (1 cup cooked)										
	11	1	1	2	0.2	0	0	0.1	38.9	7.2
Cookie, chocolate chip (1)										
	59	1	0	8	2.7	0.9	1.4	0.3	13.8	27.8
Corn (1 cup)										
	132	5	4	29	1.8	0.3	0.5	0.9	24.6	23.1
Cottage cheese, low-fat (1 cup)										
	163	28	0	6	2.3	1.5	0.7	0.1	20.3	918
Crackers (12)										
	154	3.3	1.1	25.5	4	0.6	2.5	0.4	289	781
Cranberry juice cocktail (1 cup)										
	137	0	0	34	0.3	0	0	0.1	58.2	5.1
Cream cheese (1 tbsp)										
	50	1	0	1	5	2.8	1.2	0.2	25.1	46.5
Cucumber with peel (¹⁄₂ cup)										
	8	0	0	2	0.1	0	0	0	2.6	1
Doughnut (1)										
	192	2	1	23	10.3	2.7	5.7	1.3	67	181
Egg, whole (1 large)										
	71	6	0	0	5	1.5	1.9	0.7	37	70
Eggplant (1 cup)										
	20	1	3	5	0.2	0	0	0.1	10.7	1.6
English muffin, whole-wheat (1)										
	134	6	4	27	1.4	0.2	0.3	0.6	30.4	312

Vitamin A (mcg)	Vitamin B1 (mg)	Vitamin B6 (mg)	Folate (mcg)	Vitamin C (mg)	Vitamin E (mg)	Calcium (mg)	Magnesium (mg)	Potassium (mg)	Selenium (mcg)	Zinc (mg)
20	0.05	0.01	5	0	0.83	78	26	153	2	0.83
0	0.12	0	17	0.06	0.48	10	3.6	19	5	0.1
7	0.17	0.3	31	324	0.24	85	68	1,336	1	0.41
101	0.11	0.07	41	11.25	0	71	16	366	33	1.6
~	~	~	~	~	~	20	~	~	~	~
0	0	0	0	0	0	0	0	0	0	0
0	0	0	5	0	0.05	2	5	114	0	0.02
1,542	0.08	0.24	177	35	1.67	266	38	220	1	0.5
0.04	0.01	0.01	0.9	0	0.26	2.5	3	14	0	0.06
0.26	0.06	0.16	114	12	0.15	8	44	343	1.54	1.36
25	0.05	0.15	27	0	0.02	138	11	194	20	0.86
0	0.17	0	0	0	0	28	12	48	2.4	0.2
1	0.02	0.05	0	90	0	8	5	46	0	0.18
53	0	0	2	0	0.04	12	1	17	0.4	0.1
10	0.01	0.02	7	2.76	0	7	6	75	0	0.1
17	0.1	0.03	24	0.9	0.9	21	9	60	4	0.3
84	0.03	0.06	22	0	0.5	25	5	63	15	0.5
4	0.08	0.09	14	1	0.4	6	11	122	0.1	0.12
0.09	0.25	0.05	36	0	0.26	101	21	106	17	0.61

Food	Calories	Protein	Fiber	Carbohydrate	Total Fat	Saturated Fat	Monounsaturated	Polyunsaturated	Omega 3s (mg)	Sodium (mg)
Fig bar cookies (2 bars)										
	150	2	2	30	3.1	0.5	1.3	1.2	78.3	151
Fish, white (1 fillet)										
	146	27	0	0	3.7	0.7	1.1	1.3	960	63.6
Flaxseed (1 tbsp)										
	55	2	3	3	4.3	0.4	0.8	2.9	238	3.1
French fries (10)										
	226	3	3	28	11.5	2.3	6	2.6	~	122
Fruit, dried (11 oz)										
	712	7	23	188	1.4	0.1	0.7	0.3	5.9	52.7
Garlic (1 clove)										
	4	0	0	1	0	0	0	0	0.6	0.5
Graham cracker (1 large rectangular piece)										
	59	1	0	11	1.4	0.2	0.6	0.5	36.3	84.7
Granola bar (1)										
	118	3	1	16	4.9	0.6	1.1	3	15	73.5
Grape juice (1 cup)										
	143	0	0	36	0	0	0	0	0	22.5
Grapefruit, red (½ fruit)										
	37	1	1	9	0.1	0	0	0	6.2	0
Ham (1 slice)										
	45	5	0	1	2.3	0.8	1.1	0.3	33.6	358
Hamburger, fast-food, with condiments and vegetables (1)										
	294	15	2	33	11.5	4.6	5.3	1.3	127	560
Hemp seed (2 tbsp)										
	90	5	2	3	6	1	4	1	~	0
Hot dog, fast-food (1)										
	280	11	1	22	17	6	~	~	~	710
Ice cream (1 serving)										
	137	2	0	16	7.3	4.5	2	0.3	117	52.8
Jam or preserves (1 tbsp)										
	56	0	0	14	0	0	0	0	0	6.4
Kale (1 cup)										
	33	2	1	7	0.5	0.1	0	0.2	121	28.8
Ketchup (1 tbsp)										
	15	0	0	4	0	0	0	0	0.6	167
Kiwi fruit (1 medium)										
	56	1	3	13	0.5	0	0	0.3	38.2	2.7

Vitamin A (mcg)	Vitamin B1 (mg)	Vitamin B6 (mg)	Folate (mcg)	Vitamin C (mg)	Vitamin E (mg)	Calcium (mg)	Magnesium (mg)	Potassium (mg)	Selenium (mcg)	Zinc (mg)
3	0.05	0.02	11	0.1	0.21	20	9	66	1	0.12
60	0.26	0.5	26	0	0.39	51	65	625	25	2
0	0.2	0	8.9	0.1	0	26.1	40.2	83.3	2.6	0.4
0	0.07	0.16	8	6	0.12	4	11	211	0.2	0.2
380	0.14	0.5	13	12	2	119	121	2,482	1.5	1.56
0	0	0.04	0.09	0.9	0	5	0.75	12	0.4	0
0	0.03	0.01	6	0	0.05	3	4	19	1	0.1
2	0.06	0.02	6	0.22	0.32	15	24	82	4	0.5
1	0.07	0.16	8	0.25	0	23	25	334	0.25	0.13
319	0	0.1	11.1	45.5	~	18.4	9.8	156	1.7	0.1
0	0.2	0.1	1	0	0.1	2	5	94	6	0.5
4	0.3	0.12	52	2	0.42	126	23	251	20	2
~	~	~	~	~	~	~	~	~	~	~
0	0.44	0.09	85	0.009	0.1	108	27	190	29	2
6	0.03	0.04	11	0.46	0	72	19	164	1.65	0.4
0.2	0	0	2	2	0	4	0.8	15	0.4	0
955	0.07	0.11	18	33	1	180	23	417	1.17	0.23
7	0	0.02	2	2	0.2	3	3	57	0.04	0
3	0.02	0.07	19	70	1	26	13	237	0.15	0.1

Food	Calories	Protein	Fiber	Carbohydrate	Total Fat	Saturated Fat	Monounsaturated	Polyunsaturated	Omega 3s (mg)	Sodium (mg)
Lasagna, meat (7 oz)										
	377	25	4	38	14	6.7	5.3	1	116	832
Lentils (1 tbsp)										
	42	3	4	7	0.1	0	0	0.1	13.1	0.7
Lettuce, iceberg (1 cup)										
	10	1	1	2	0.1	0	0	0.1	37.4	7.2
Lettuce, romaine (½ cup)										
	8	1	1	2	0.1	0	0	0.1	53.1	3.8
Liver, beef (3 oz)										
	114	18	0	3	3	1	0.3	0.3	2	19.3
Lunch meat, salami (3 slices)										
	99	7	0	0	7.7	3	4.1	0.8	71	534
Macaroni and cheese (8 oz)										
	259	11	1	48	2.6	1.3	~	~	~	561
Meat loaf (1 slice)										
	205	20	0	0	13.1	5.3	6.3	0.4	12.7	62
Melon, honeydew (1 cup)										
	64	1	1	16	0.2	0.1	0	0.1	58.4	31.9
Milk, fat-free (1 cup)										
	83	8	0	12	0.2	0.1	0.1	0	2.5	103
Milk, soy (1 cup)										
	100	7	1	8	4	0.5	0	0	~	119
Muffin, blueberry (1)										
	181	3	3	36	3	1.1	0.6	1	107	224
Mushrooms (1 cup sliced)										
	15	2	1	2	0.2	0	0	0.1	~	3.5
Nachos with cheese (6–8)										
	346	9	~	36	18.9	7.8	8	2.2	195	816
Nectarine (1)										
	63	2	2	15	0.5	0	0.1	0.2	2.9	0
Oatmeal (1 cup, cooked)										
	150	5	4	28	3	0.5	0.8	0.9	40	2.5
Olive oil, extra-virgin (1 tbsp)										
	119	0	0	0	13.5	1.9	9.8	1.4	103	0.3
Olives (1 tbsp)										
	9	0	0	1	0.9	0.1	0.7	0.1	5.3	71.9
Onion rings (10 medium)										
	276	4	~	31	15.5	7	6.7	0.7	107	430

Vitamin A (mcg)	Vitamin B1 (mg)	Vitamin B6 (mg)	Folate (mcg)	Vitamin C (mg)	Vitamin E (mg)	Calcium (mg)	Magnesium (mg)	Potassium (mg)	Selenium (mcg)	Zinc (mg)
61	0.19	0.2	16	12	0.94	220	41	372	28	3
0.05	0.02	0.01	57.5	0.5	0.1	6.7	14.6	115	1.0	0.6
8	0.02	0.03	31	2	0.02	11	4	84	0.28	0.1
81	0.02	0.02	38	7	0.04	9	4	69	0.1	0.06
8,042	0.16	0.86	215	1.62	0.43	5	18	300	31	4.5
0	0.1	0.08	0.34	0	0.05	1.34	2.86	63	4	0.54
48	0.25	0	0	0	0	102	0	111	0	0
20	0.1	0.14	12	0.62	0.1	43	22	295	0	4
5	0.07	0.16	34	32	0.04	11	18	403	1.24	0.16
5	0.1	0.1	12	2	0.1	301	27	406	5	1
0	0.15	0.16	40	0	0	80	60	440	3	0.9
13	0.1	0.01	42	2	0.1	5	10	355	8	0.7
0	0.09	0.1	12	2	0.1	5	10	355	8	0.7
170	0.2	0.2	12	1	0	311	63	196	18	2
23	0.05	0.03	7	7	1	8	12	273	0	0.23
0.12	0.12	0.1	13	0	0.26	19	51	175	0	1.43
0	0	0	0	0	1.9	0.1	0	0.1	0	0
1.7	0	0	0	0	0.14	7	0.3	0.67	0.08	0
0.98	0.1	0.07	64	0.68	0.39	86	19	152	3	0.41

Food	Calories	Protein	Fiber	Carbohydrate	Total Fat	Saturated Fat	Monounsaturated	Polyunsaturated	Omega 3s (mg)	Sodium (mg)
Oyster (1 medium)										
	41	5	0	2	1.1	0.3	0.2	0.4	370	53
Pancakes (2)										
	172	4	~	22	7.4	1.6	1.8	3.4	196	167
Pasta (4 oz, cooked)										
	150	6	~	28	2	1.2	0.2	0.2	42.2	6.8
Peach (1 medium)										
	68	2	3	17	0.4	0	0.1	0.2	3.5	0
Peanut butter (2 tbsp)										
	188	8	2	6	16.1	3.4	7.7	4.5	25	147
Peanuts (1 oz)										
	159	7	2	5	13.8	1.9	6.8	4.4	0.8	5
Pear (1 medium)										
	61	1	5	14	0.8	0.1	0.1	0.3	34.3	7.5
Pepper, chile, raw (1/2 pepper)										
	18	1	1	4	0.2	0	0	0.1	5	4
Peppers, sweet (10 strips)										
	14	1	0	3	0.1	0	~	~	~	1
Pie, apple (1 piece)										
	296	2	2	42	13.8	4.7	5.5	2.7	154	332
Pizza, cheese (1 slice)										
	272	12	2	34	9.8	4.3	2.4	1.8	174	551
Plum (1)										
	30	0	1	8	0.2	0	0.1	0	~	0
Popcorn (1 cup)										
	31	1	1	6	0.4	0	0.1	0.2	4.8	0.6
Pork (3 oz)										
	90	18	0	0	3	0.6	0.6	0.3	2	68
Potato salad (1 cup)										
	324	3	~	39	18	3	4.8	8.7	855	936
Potatoes, mashed (1 cup)										
	174	4	3	37	1.2	0.5	0.2	0.1	35.7	634
Pot pie, chicken										
	380	11	3	36	21.5	8.3	9.2	3.7	~	841
Pretzels (10 twists)										
	227	6	2	48	1.6	0.3	0.7	0.7	44.4	814
Quinoa (1 cup, cooked)										
	222	8	5	39	3.6	~	~	~	~	13

Vitamin A (mcg)	Vitamin B₁ (mg)	Vitamin B₆ (mg)	Folate (mcg)	Vitamin C (mg)	Vitamin E (mg)	Calcium (mg)	Magnesium (mg)	Potassium (mg)	Selenium (mcg)	Zinc (mg)
4.2	0.01	0.01	1.4	0.52	0.12	6	7	22	9	13
7.6	0.16	0.07	28	0.15	0.65	96	15	133	10	0.3
0	0.13	0.1	4	6	1.4	41	13	207	11	0.66
16	0.02	0.02	4	6	0.7	6	9	186	0.1	0.17
0	0.03	0.15	24	0	0	12	51	214	2	1
0	0.12	0.07	41	0	2	15	50	186	2	1
1.6	0.02	0.05	12	7	0.2	15	12	198	0.17	0.17
21.6	0.03	0.23	10.35	65	0.3	6	10	145	0.2	0.12
78	0.04	0.13	13	70	0.036	7	6.46	105	0	0
37	0.03	0.04	32	4	1.78	13	8	76	1	0.2
74	0.2	0.04	35	1	0	117	16	113	13	1
21	0.03	0.05	1.45	6	0	3	5	114	0.3	0.07
0.8	0.02	0.02	2	0	0	1	11	24	0.8	0.3
~	0.8	0.3	3	0	0.2	6	15	253	14	2
2.93	0.2	0.4	19	19	0.14	14	36	551	10	0.6
8.4	0.2	0.5	17	13	0.04	46	38	621	2	0.6
256	0.3	0.2	41	2	4	33	24	256	0.7	1
0	0.3	0.07	103	0	0.21	22	21	88	3	0.5
9.3	0.2	0.2	77.7	0	1.2	31.5	118	318	5.2	2

Food	Calories	Protein	Fiber	Carbohydrate	Total Fat	Saturated Fat	Monounsaturated	Polyunsaturated	Omega 3s (mg)	Sodium (mg)
Raisins (1½ oz)										
	129	1	2	34	0.2	0	0	0	3	4.7
Raspberries (10)										
	10	0	1	2	0.1	0	0	0.1	23.9	0.2
Rice, brown (1 cup, cooked)										
	216	5	4	45	1.8	0.4	0.6	0.6	27.3	9.8
Rice, white (1 cup)										
	242	4	1	53	0.4	0.1	0.1	0.1	18.6	0
Ricotta cheese, part skim (½ cup)										
	171	14	0	6	9.8	6.1	2.9	0.3	86.8	155
Salad dressing, light Italian (1 tbsp)										
	28	0	0	1	2.8	0.4	0.7	1.6	190	199
Salmon (3 oz)										
	177	17	0	0	11.4	2.6	3.2	3.3	2,130	50.1
Salsa (½ cup)										
	35	2	2	8	0.2	0	0	0.1	6.5	780
Sardines (1 can)										
	191	23	0	0	10.5	1.4	3.6	4.7	1,362	465
Sauerkraut (1 cup)										
	31	1	4	6	0.1	0	0	0.1	35.5	437
Sausage (1 link)										
	286	16	0	4	22.7	7.9	9.9	2.7	365	1,002
Shrimp (4 large)										
	30	6	0	0	0.5	0.1	0.1	0.2	151	41.4
Soft drink with caffeine (12 oz)										
	136	0	0	35	0.1	0	0	0	0	14.7
Soup, cream of chicken (1 cup)										
	120	3	2	10	8	2.5	~	~	~	870
Soup, tomato (1 cup)										
	91	2	1	20	0	0	0	0	0	710
Soybeans (1 cup cooked)										
	298	29	10	17	15.4	2.2	3.4	8.7	1,029	1.7
Spare ribs (3 oz)										
	303	18	0	0	25.8	7.8	9	2.4	104.1	76.5
Spinach (1 cup)										
	7	1	1	1	0.1	0	0	0	41.4	23.7
Steak (3 oz)										
	159	18	0	0	9.3	3.9	3.9	0.3	111.6	44.4

Vitamin A (mcg)	Vitamin B1 (mg)	Vitamin B6 (mg)	Folate (mcg)	Vitamin C (mg)	Vitamin E (mg)	Calcium (mg)	Magnesium (mg)	Potassium (mg)	Selenium (mcg)	Zinc (mg)
0	0.05	0.08	1.28	2.3	0.3	12	13	350	0.26	0.08
0.38	0.01	0.01	4	5	0.17	5	4	28	0.04	0.08
0	0.2	0.3	8	0	0.06	20	84	84	19	1
0	0.03	0.15	5	0	0.06	16	19	55	12	0.8
132	0.03	0.02	16	0	0.09	337	19	155	21	1.7
0	0	0	0	0	0	0	0	2	0.2	0
9.84	0.2	0.71	22	0	0.95	11	28	475	35	0.6
44	0.05	0.16	21	18	1.53	39	17	275	0.5	0.3
99.3	0.1	0.2	11	0	1.9	351	35.9	365	48.5	1.2
1.42	0.03	0.18	34	21	0.14	43	18	241	0.9	0.3
0	0.05	0.01	0.26	0	0.03	1.3	1.56	25	1.87	0.24
0	0.01	0.03	0.77	0.48	0	9	7	40	9	0.3
0	0	0	0	0	0	10	3	3	0.34	0
179	0.07	0.07	7	1.24	0.25	181	17	272	8	0.67
29.28	0.09	0.11	15	66	2	12	7	263	0.5	0.24
14	0.47	0.1	200	31	0.02	261	108	970	3	1.64
1.91	0.26	0.22	3	0	0.2	30	15	204	24	3
140	0.02	0.06	58	8	0.6	30	24	167	0.3	0.16
0	0.1	0.3	6	0	0.11	4	19	250	12	3.26

Food	Calories	Protein	Fiber	Carbohydrate	Total Fat	Saturated Fat	Monounsaturated	Polyunsaturated	Omega 3s (mg)	Sodium (mg)
Strawberries (1 cup)										
	49	1	3	12	0.5	0	0.1	0.2	98.8	1.5
Submarine sandwich										
	456	22	~	51	18.6	6.8	8.2	2.3	~	1,651
Sweet potato (1)										
	112	2	4	26	0.1	0	0	0	1.3	71.5
Taco salad (1½ cups)										
	279	13	~	24	14.8	6.8	5.2	1.7	89.1	762
Toaster pastry (1)										
	209	2	1	37	5.6	1.3	3.3	0.7	37.2	181
Tofu (½ cup)										
	183	20	3	5	11	1.6	2.4	6.2	733	17.6
Tomato (1 medium)										
	32	2	1	6	0.6	0.1	0.1	0.2	8.5	48.8
Tuna salad (1 cup)										
	383	33	0	19	19	3.2	5.9	8.5	822	824
Vegetable juice (1 cup)										
	46	2	2	11	0.2	0	0	0.1	2.4	653
Walnuts (1 oz)										
	183	4	2	4	18.3	1.7	2.5	13.2	2,542	0.6
Watermelon (1 wedge)										
	86	2	1	22	0.4	0	0.1	0.1	~	2.9
Wine, red (3½ oz)										
	88	0	0	3.5	0	0	0	0	0	~
Wine, white (3½ oz)										
	84	0	0	3.4	0	0	0	0	0	5.25
Yogurt, low-fat (8 oz)										
	238	11	0	42	3.2	2.1	0.9	0.1	27.2	132

Vitamin A (mcg)	Vitamin B₁ (mg)	Vitamin B₆ (mg)	Folate (mcg)	Vitamin C (mg)	Vitamin E (mg)	Calcium (mg)	Magnesium (mg)	Potassium (mg)	Selenium (mcg)	Zinc (mg)
1.66	0.03	0.09	40	97	0.5	27	22	253	1	0.2
71	1	0.1	87	12	0	189	68	394	31	2.6
350	0.09	0.25	9	19	1.42	41	27	348	0.3	0.3
176	0.1	0.2	83	4	~	192	51	416	4.4	2.7
148	0.2	0.2	15	0	0.9	17	12	57	6.3	0.3
4.96	0.1	0.06	19	0	0.01	434	37	150	11	1
26	0.02	0.05	9	8	0.33	6	7	146	0	0.11
49	0.06	0.17	16	5	2	35	39	365	84	1
188	0.1	0.3	51	67	12	26	27	467	1	0.5
5.6	0.1	0.2	27.4	0.4	0.2	27.4	44.2	123	1.4	0.9
104	0.2	0.4	6	31	0.4	41	31	479	0.3	0.2
0	0	0.03	2	0	0	8	13	111	0.2	0.1
0	0	0.01	0	0	0	9	10	80	0.2	0.07
2	0.1	0.09	24	1.7	0	415	37	497	11	1.88

ACKNOWLEDGMENTS

This book would not have been possible without the support, guidance, and hard work of the following:

Gina Centrello, Bill Takes, Libby McGuire, Marnie Cochran, Jennie Tung, Richard Callison, Joe Perez, Nina Shield, Susan Corcoran, Theresa Zoro, Cindy Murry, Sanyu Dillon, Kristin Fassler, and Quinne Rogers at Ballantine.

Stephen Perrine, George Karabotsos, Cecelia Smith, Michael Freidson, Ray Jobst, Sean Bumgarner, Jon Hammond, Charlene Lutz, Kimberly Miller, Linh Le, Daniel Cohen, and the entire team at Galvanized.

Master chef Matt Goulding.

Researchers Heather Hurlock and Wendy Hess; fitness gurus Shawn Perine and Sean Hyson; and many others who contributed to this effort.

The teams at *Good Morning America* and *ABC News,* who have supported my efforts at every turn.

Jennifer Rudolph Walsh, Jon Rosen, Andy McNichol, and the brilliant minds at WME.

Larry Shire, Eric Sacks, and Jonathan Ehrlich, for their invaluable counsel.

Mehmet Oz, David Pecker, Dave Freygang, Strauss Zelnick, Joe Armstrong, Dan Abrams, Michele Promaulayko, and the many friends, colleagues, and advisers who continue to inspire me with their wisdom and insight.

And the best family a man could ever be blessed with.

INDEX

water intake, 103–4
"spa water," 262
during workouts, 155
in ZERO BELLY cleanse, 262, 264
watermelon, 73
weight cycling, 257–58
weight loss:
healthy gut bacteria and, 37–38
long-term, fast results and,
258–59
7 habits for success in, 108–9
teas that speed, 268–69
wheat, gluten and, xxvii, 44, 75
whey protein, 78
white fat, 47
browning of, 46–47
white tea, 269
Who You Callin' Chicken Burger, 142
William Paterson University, 81
Wilson, Bryan, xxiv, 96, 111
Wilson, Russell, 54–55, 59–60
Windshield Wiper, 249
Wood Chop, 214
workouts, ZERO BELLY, xxv, xxvii,
109, 149–254
Barbell, 166–73
Dumbell, 174–81
eating schedule and, 97, 98
Full-Body Challenge, 156–65
at a glance, xxvii
HIIT Body-Weight, 194–200
Kettlebell, 201–5

Medicine Ball, 216–23
metabolic circuits and, 153–55
Suspension, 182–93
Swiss Ball, 206–15
10-Minute Snaxercize Circuit,
254
see also Seven-Minute Abs
Workouts, ZERO BELLY
World Health Organization, 27

yogurt, 42, 44, 45

ZERO BELLY at a Glance, xxvi–xxvii
ZERO BELLY cleanse, *see* Seven-Day
Cleanse, ZERO BELLY
ZERO BELLY foods, xxvi
see also ingredients, ZERO
BELLY
ZERO BELLY guidelines, *see*
guidelines for ZERO BELLY
ZERO BELLY recipes, *see* breakfasts,
ZERO BELLY; burgers, ZERO
BELLY; drinks, ZERO BELLY;
lunches, ZERO BELLY, dinners,
ZERO BELLY; snacks, ZERO
BELLY
ZERO BELLY workouts, *see* Seven-
Minute Abs Workouts, ZERO
BELLY; workouts, ZERO BELLY
zucchini:
Skinny Thai, 132
Voodoo Chili, 125

ABOUT THE AUTHOR

DAVID ZINCZENKO is the *New York Times* bestselling co-author (with Matt Goulding) of the Eat This, Not That! series (which has sold more than eight million copies in North America), the Abs Diet books, *The 8-Hour Diet,* and most recently *Eat It to Beat It!* He is the award-winning former editor in chief of *Men's Health* and editorial director of *Women's Health, Prevention,* and *Best Life* magazines. He's ABC News's nutrition and wellness editor and special correspondent; he is also editorial director of *Men's Fitness* and *Shape* and CEO of the media company Galvanized LLC. He lives in New York City.

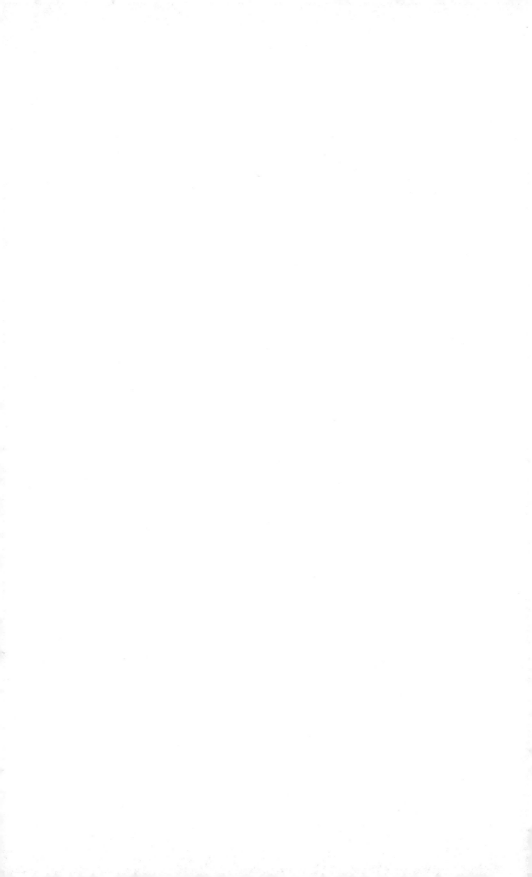